Evidence-Based Reflexology Research for Health Professionals and Researchers

The Reflexology Research Series

Key to symbols used in this document
Throughout this work, specific studies are cited in the text. They are identified with a number in parentheses, i. e. (21). (A full Bibliography of the numbered studies begins on page 202.) Also cited is further information about the study. The information is represented by symbols, i. e. (21)*•. Represented by symbols are: a controlled study*; a PubMed listed study•; a study published in a Korean peer-reviewed journal^; a study published in a Chinese peer-reviewed journal+.

Thus, a citation of (21)*• is a controlled study listed with PubMed, specifically:
 (21)*• Stephenson NL, Swanson M, Dalton J, Keefe FJ, Engelke M. "Partner-delivered reflexology: effects on cancer pain and anxiety," *Oncology Nursing Forum* 2007 Jan;34(1):127-32.

* Indicates a Controlled study
• Indicates a PubMed listed study (National Institute of Health)
^ Indicates a study published in a Korean peer-reviewed journal
+ Indicates a study published in a Chinese peer-reviewed journal

Also available in The Reflexology Research Documents Series:
Evidence-Based Reflexology Research for You and Your Family (51 pages)
Evidence-Based Reflexology Research for Reflexologists (84 pages)

Reflexology Research Project, P. O. Box 35820, Albuquerque, NM 87107
e-mail: footc@mac.com • Phone: 505-344-9392

© Kunz & Kunz 2008 All rights reserved. No part of this book may be reproduced in any form or by any means without permission in writing from the publisher.

Reflexology is not intended to be a substitute for medical care. If you have a health problem, consult a medical professional.

Web Sites hosted by Kunz & Kunz
www.reflexology-research.com
www.foot-reflexologist.com
www.myreflexologist.com

Books by Barbara and Kevin Kunz
The Complete Guide to Foot Reflexology (1980); (Revised) (1993); (Third Edition, 2005)
Hand And Foot Reflexology, A Self-help Guide (Simon & Schuster) (1984)
Hand Reflexology Workbook, How to work on someone's hands (1985); (Revised, 1999)
The Parent's Guide to Reflexology (HarperCollins) (1997)
Medical Applications of Reflexology / RRP Press (1999); (Revised, 2003)
My Reflexologist Says Feet Don't Lie / RRP Press (2001)
Reflexology: Health at Your Fingertips / DK (2003)
Hand Reflexology / DK (2006)
Complete Reflexology for Life / DK (2007)
Total Reflexology (Kit) / Barnes & Noble (2007)
The Reflexology Path / Barnes & Noble (2009)

Table of Contents (In Brief)

Introduction   20

Chapter One: Factors Impacting Successful Outcomes and Research   21

Chapter Two: What Reflexology Research Demonstrates   32

Chapter Three: Procedures and Outcomes for 169 Studies and 78 Disorders / Physical Conditions   46

Chapter Four: Physiologic Measures, Dosing and Results   117

Chapter Five: Effects on Physiological Processes 129

Chapter Six: Systems of the Body, Dosing and Results   136

Chapter Seven: Formula for Reflexology Dosing as Shown by Research 141

Chapter Eight: Benchmarks for Dosing and Results   167

Chapter Nine: Formula for Hand Reflexology, Self-Help Reflexology, Self-Help Tool Use   177

Chapter Ten: Discussion of Negative Outcomes   182

Chapter Eleven: Control Groups: Impact on Outcomes   198

Bibliography   206

Table of Contents / Research Index

Introduction 20

Chapter One: Creating Successful Outcomes and Research 21

Technique Application: Its role in successful outcomes 22
- Frequency (How often technique is applied) 22
- Duration of reflexology session   22
- Amount of pressure / Intensity   23
- Reflexology method   24
- Mode of technique delivery (Foot reflexology, Hand reflexology, Self-help reflexology)   24

- Reflex areas (Where technique is applied)   25
- The human variable: the client, the reflexologist and the medical practitioner   25
- Impact of multiple factors   26
- Cultural and historic factors   26

Interpreting Efficacy: Evaluating performance 27
- Reporting of results: Its importance in clarifying outcomes   27
- Quantitative vs. Qualitative Measures (Patient's view vs. objective measures) 28
- Timing of measurement 29
- Blinding 29

(*See also: Chapter Ten: Discussion of Negative Outcomes, page 179*)

Control Groups: Impact on outcomes   30
- Use of sham or placebo reflexology as a control   30
- Use of foot massage as a control   31

(*See also: Chapter Eleven: Control Groups: Impact on Outcomes, page 194*)

Chapter Two: What Reflexology Research Demonstrates   32

Summary of results   33
Impact on specific organs 33
Amelioration of symptoms   34
Creation of a relaxation effect   35
Aid to pain reduction   36
Impact on physiological measures   38
Improvement in blood flow   41
Beneficial for post-operative recovery and pain reduction   41
Enhancement of medical care   42
Adjunct to mental health care 42
Complement to cancer care   44
Easier birthing / delivery   44

Chapter Three: Procedures and Outcomes for 168 Studies and 78 Disorders / Physical Conditions   46

A Page 47
Aggressive, anti-social behavior in children (Mainstreaming) (135)
AIDS (Pain and fatigue) (42)*
Anxiety, salivary cortisol and melatonin (41)*•
Appetite *See Cancer (Quality of life) (151)•; Hospice (136)*; Athletes (153)*+ ; Postpartum women (159)*+*
Arthritis (43)+
Asthma (44)*•
Asthma (142)*+
Asthma (139)*•
Asthma (45)*•

B *Page 49*
Birthing / Delivery
  Labor outcomes (45)*•
  Pain killing (47)*
  Labor outcomes (46)
  Relieving labor pains (48)
  Primary inertia (165)*
  Recovering gastointestinal functioon after Cesarean section (163)*+
  See also Postpartum women
Blood pressure
  Senior citizens (25)*•
  Baroreceptor reflex sensitivity, blood pressure and sinus arrhythmia (26)*
  Healthy individuals (41)*•
  Coronary heart disease (30)*+
  Middle aged women (3)*•^
  Nursing home residents with dementia (31)*•
  Hypertension (11)*•^
  Hypertension in the elderly (8)*^
  Senior citizens (28)•
  Coronary artery bypass graft patients (29)*•
  Hypertension (58)*

C *Page 54*
Cancer
  Chemotherapy (Blood pressure, pulse, fatigue, mood, foot fatigue (5)*^
  Chemotherapy (Nausea, vomiting, fatigue) (4)*•^
  Chemotherapy (Nausea, vomiting) (158)*+
  Radiotherapy (Fatigue, anxiety, mood) (152)*
  Psycho-neuroimmunoloical response (168)*
  Pain and nausea (22)•
  Pain and anxiety (21)*•
  Pain / Anxiety) (134)•
  Anxiety (second and third round of chemotherapy)) (23)*•
  Fatigue (advanced cancer) (24)•
  Pain (57)•
  Quality of life (151)•
  Pain and anxiety following surgery (157)*
  Depression, anxiety, quality of life, spirituality (140)
Cerebral palsy (Growth rates) (49)*+
Cervical spondylosis (Degeneration of cervical vertebrae or pad between vertebrae)(116)*+
Cervical spondylosis (122)+
Cervical spondylosis (Free radicals) (50)+
Cholesterol (Hypertensioon in the elderly) (8)*^
Cholesterol and triglycerides in the blood (Hyperlipimia)(84)*
Cholesterol and monoglyceride (Hyperlipimia)(85)+
Cholesterol (Menopausal women) (12)*^
Cholesterol (Hypertension (58)*

Chronic fatigue syndrome (153)
Chronic obstructive pulmonary disorder (COPD) (149)*•
Circulation (Foot) (120)+
Circulation (Peripheral blood circulation) (Diabetes mellitus (type 2) (6)*^
Circulation (Foot), Temperature, Galvanic skin response (104)
Colic (138)
Constipation (Elderly and healthy volunteers)(59)*+
Constipation (Middle-aged women)(60)
Constipation (Children) (61)*

D *Page 65*

Deafness (Loss of hearing due to drug toxic effects) (117)+
Dementia (Efficacy as a Palliative Treatment in Nursing Home Residents with Dementia) (31)*•
Diabetes mellitus (type 2)
  Peripheral blood circulation, Peripheral neuropathy) (6)*^
  Fasting glucose levels (33)*•+
  Blood flow to the feet (35)*
  Fasting glucose levels (34)*+
  Pulse, fatigue, mood (7)*^
Diagnosis (145)•
Diagnosis (146)
Diagnosis (147)
Doppler sonogram (Kidney) (69)*•
Doppler sonogram (Intestines)(68)*•
Doppler (Circulation in Diabetes mellitus (type 2)) (35)*
Dyspepsia (83)+

E *Page 69*

ECG (71)
ECG Heart rate variability) (63)
ECG (Coronary heart disease) (30)*+
ECG (Angina) (62)+
Edema (Pregnancy) (148)*•
EEG (64)
EEG (65)•
EEG (66)•
EEG (70)
EEG (Physiological measurement) (137)
Encopresis (Fecal incontinence)/ Chronic constipation (90)*•
Enuresis (52)*•
Enuresis (154)
Enuresis (126)+
Epilepsy (91)+

F *Page 75*

fMRI (Vision) (128)
fMRI (Adrenal gland reflex area stimulation compared to acupuncture K1 (comparable acupoint)) (129)
fMRI (Temporal lobe activation) (127)

fMRI (Eye, shoulder, small intestines) (169)
Fatigue and sleep (Nurses) (9)*^
Fatigue (Athletes) (53)*+
Free radicals (Cervical spondylosis) (50)*+
Free radicals (51)*+
G *Page 77*
Gout (115)*+
H *Page 77*
Headaches (92)
Hemodialysis (10)*^
Hemodialysis and Cancer (40)*
Hemodialysis (Cramping) (155)
Hepatitis B (118)+
Herniated disc/lumbro-sacral (Pain) (72)•
Herpes zoster (114)+
Hospice (136)*•
Hospice (80)•
Hyperlipimia (Cholesterol and triglycerides in the blood)(84)*
Hyperlipimia (Cholesterol and monoglyceride)(85)+
Hypertension in the elderly (8)*^
Hypertension (11)*•^
Hypertension (58)*
I *Page 81*
Immune System (Hemodialysis) (10)*^
Immune System (Depression, Stress Responses, Immune Functions /Middle Aged Women) (3)*•^
Incontinence in middle-aged women (17)*^
Incontinence in middle-aged women (36)*•
Infertility (84)*
Infertility / Ovulation (164)*
Insomnia (54) (*See also Sleep*)
Insomnia (87)*+ (*See also Sleep*)
Irritable bowel (56)
Irritable bowel (55)*•
K *Page 84*
Kidney stones (74)*
Kidney function (69)*
Kidney and ureter stones (Recovery from lithotrity) (78)*+
Knee replacement (Recovery from surgery) (141)*
L *Page 86*
Lactation in new mothers (96)*+
Leukopenia (Pathologically low white blood cell count) (121)*+
Lower back pain (93)*
Lower back pain (Chronic) (105)*
M *Page 88*
Menopausal women (37)*•
Menopausal women (89)+

Menopausal women (12)*^
Mental health (88)
Mental health (150)
Mental retardation (95)*+
Middle-aged women (3)*•^
Migraine headache (94)*
Migraine headache (130)
Multiple sclerosis (97)*
Multiple sclerosis (98)*
Multiple sclerosis (167)
Myopia (123)+
Myopia (Adolescent) (119)+

N *Page 95*
Nervous exhaustion (100)
Neurodermatitis (99)*+
Neuropathy (Diabetes, Type 2) (6)*^

O *Page 96*
Osteoarthritis (13)*^
Osteoarthritis (144)*
Ovulation (164)*
Oxygen saturation, Pulse rate, Respiratory rate (124)+

P *Page 97*
Pain
  Threshold and tolerance (75)
  Palliative Treatment in Nursing Home Residents with Dementia (31)*•
  Pain (Miscellaneous) (76)+
  AIDS (42)*
  Birthing/Relieving labor pains (47)*
  Birthing/ Relieving labor pains (48)
  Blood pressure, pain, control over falls in senior citizens (25)*•
  Cancer/Pain and anxiety (21)*•
  Cancer/Pain and nausea (22)•
  Cancer/Pain (57)•
  Cancer / Pain management / Anxiety (134)•
  Chest pain (73)
  Diabetes mellitus (type 2) Peripheral blood circulation, Peripheral neuropathy)(6)*^
  Herniated disc/lumbro-sacral (72)•
  Kidney stones (74)*
  Lower back (Chronic) (105)*
  Lower back (93)*
  Osteoarthritis (13)*^
  Phantom limb (67) •
  Post operative / General surgery (101)*
  Post operative / Cancer patients (157)*
  Post surgical / Prostatectomy (143)*•
  Post operative / Gynecological (82)*

(Post) Surgical ward (172)
  Post surgical / Abdominal (81)*•
  Post surgical / Open heart (106)*
  Post surgical / Knee replacement (141)*
  Premenstrual syndrome/ Dysmenorrhea (15)*^
  Sinusitis (77)*
Peptic ulcers (156)*+
Phantom limb pain (67)•
Physiological measure (137)
Pneumoconiosis (Coal workers') (2)*•^
Pneumoconiosis (Coal workers') (1)*^
Pneumonia (102)+
Polycystic ovaries (103)
Postpartum women
  Post-partum women recovering from Cesarean section (Gastrointestinal function)(163)*
  Postpartum women (160)*+
  Post partum (159)*+
  Postpartum women (Anxiety and depression) (161)*+
  Postpartum women (14)*^
Post surgical
  Pain / General surgery (101)*
  Pain and anxiety among cancer patients (157)*
  Pain / elderly patients following prostatectomy (143)*
  Post surgical recovery (107)*
  Recovery (Abdominal) (81)*
  Recovery (Gynecological) (82)*
Post traumatic stress disorder (133)
Post traumatic stress disorder (132)
Premature infants (162)*+
Premenstrual syndrome (38)*•
Premenstrual syndrome/ Dysmenorrhea (15)*^
Prostate (108)
Prostate (Hyperplasia)(110)*+
Prostate (Hypertrophy) (109)+

S *Page 113*
Sinusitis (77)*
Sleep
  Sleep disturbance, depression disorder, and the physiological index) (39)*•+
  Elderly women (16)*^
  Pneumoconiosis (coal workers') (2)*•^
  Fatigue (Nurses) (9)*^
  Insomnia (87)*+
Stress (Mothers staying with hospitalized children) (166)
Stroke (18)*^
Stroke (125)+
Students (Constipation, anxiety, depression) (19)*^

T *Page 116*
Thyroid (171)
U *Page 116*
Urinary tract infection (112)*+
Urinary tract stones (Lithotrity) (78)*+
Urinary tract stones (111)+
Uroshesis (113)*+
W *White blood cell count See Leukopenia*

Chapter Four: Physiologic Measures, Dosing and Results 117

Alpha amyase (31)
Blood Pressure
  Senior citizens (25)*•
  Coronary heart disease patients (30)*+
  Hypertensive patients (11)*•^
  Nursing home residents (31)*•
  Healthy volunteers (137)
  Elderly with hypertension (8)*^
  Senior citizens (28)•
  Healthy individuals (26)*
Blood Pressure (Systolic)
  Healthy volunteers (41)*•
  Cancer patients/chemotherapy (5)*^
  Cancer patients/chemotherapy (42)*
  Elderly with hypertension (8)*^
  Coronary artery bypass patients (29)*•
  Coronary heart disease patients (30)*+
  Cancer (152)*
  Middle-aged women (3)*•^
  Hypertensive patients (11)*•^
Blood Pressure (Diastolic)
  Cancer patients/chemotherapy (42)*
  Cancer patients/chemotherapy (5)*^
  Coronary heart disease patients (30)*+
  Healthy individuals (41)*•
  Hypertension in the elderly (8)*^
  Coronary artery bypass patients (29)*•
  Cancer (152)*
  Senior citizens (25)*•
  Middle-aged women (3)*•^
  Hypertensive patients (11)*•^
Blood uric acid level (115)*+
Carbon dioxide (exhaled) (137)
Carbon dioxide density (137)
Cholesterol (83)+; (84)*; (85)+; (8)*^

Cortisol (31)*•; (41)*•; (3)*•^; (167); (168)*
Doppler sonogram (35)*; (68)*•; (69)*•
ECG (30)*+; (137); (62)+; (63)
EEG (64); (66)•; (137); (65)•
fMRI (127); (128); (129) (169)
Free radicals (51)*+; (50)*+
Human growth hormone (168)*
Immune system (10)*^; (40)*; (3)*•^
Intestinal function (69)*
Kidney function (68)*•; (40)*; (10)*^
Melatonin (41)*•
Oxygen density (137)
Pancreas function (35)*; (33)*•+; (34)*+
Prolactin (168)*
Pulse rate (41)*•; (31)*•; (42)*; (137); (28)•; (30)*+; (40)*; (152)*; (3)*•^
Serotonin (39)*•+
Triglycerides (11)*•^; (14)*^; (83)+; (8)*^; (12)*^; (58)*; (11)*•^
Uric acid (115)*+
White blood cell count (121)*+

Chapter Five: Effects on Physiologic Processes 129

Doppler: (68)*•; (69)*•; (35)*
fMRI: (127); (128); (129) (169)
ECG: (63); ECG (71)
EEG: (64); (65)•; (66)•;EEG (70)
Pain (Threshold and tolerance:) (75)

Chapter Six: Systems of the Body, Dosing and Results 136

Cardio vascular system (41)*•; (28)•; (151)•; (30)*+; (31)*•; (5)*^; (8)*^; (29)*•; (3)*•^; (42)*; (5)*^; (30)*+; (29)*•; (25)*•; (3)*•^; (11)*•^; (3)*•^

Digestive system (68)*•; (59)*+; (61)*; (60); (84)*; (11); (8); 12); (58)*; (115)*+; (156)*+

Endocrine system (33)*•+; (34); (7)*^:(Reproductive System) (47)*; (46); (45)* (89)+; (12)*^; (37)*•; (103); (163)*; (159)*+; (158)*; (160)*+; (14)*^; (15)*^; (108)

Immune system (10)*^; (40)*; (3)*•^; (121)*+

Nervous system (64); (65)•; (66)•; (127); (128); (129; (97)*;. (98)*; (18)*^; (125)+

Respiratory system (142)*+; (139)*•; (44)*•; Increased (124)+; (102)+; Impacted (124)+

Skeletal system (141)* (93)*;(105)*; (13)*^; (144)*; (67)•

Urinary system (109)+; (52)*•; (154); (126)+; (17)*^; (36)*•

Chapter Seven: Formula for Results: Reflexology Dosing as Shown by Research 141

Alphabetical list of 78 disorders and physical concerns with frequency of technique application and results

A *Page 142*
Aggressive, anti-social behavior in children (137)
AIDS (Pain and fatigue) (42)*
Anxiety
  Healthy individuals (41)*•
  Cancer patients post operatively (157)*
  Cancer patients (Partner delivered) (21)*•
  Cancer: second and third round of chemotherapy (23)*•
  Pneumoconiosis (1)*^
  Cancer (134)•
  Student nurses (19)*^
  Palliative care patients (80)•
  Coronary Artery Bypass Graft) (29)*•
  Menopausal women (37)*•
Arthritis (Shoulder/acromioclaviclar) (43)+
Asthma (44)*•; (142)*; (139)*•

B *Page 143*
Birthing / Delivery
  Labor time (48)
  Pain killing (47)*
  Analgesia use (46)
  Pain killing (45)*•
  Lactation (96)*+
  Primary inertia (165)*
Blood Pressure
  Coronary heart disease patients (30)*+
  Hypertensive patients (11)*•^
  Nursing home residents (31)*•
  Healthy volunteers (137)
  Elderly with hypertension (8)*^
  Senior citizens (28)•
  Healthy individuals (26)*
  Senior citizens (25)*•
Blood Pressure (Systolic)
  Healthy volunteers (41)*•
  Cancer patients/chemotherapy (5)*^
  Cancer patients/chemotherapy (42)*
  Elderly with hypertension (8)*^
  Coronary artery bypass patients (29)*•
  Coronary heart disease patients (30)*+
  Cancer (152)*

Middle-aged women (3)*•^
  Hypertensive patients (11)*•^
Blood Pressure (Diastolic)
  Cancer patients/chemotherapy (42)*
  Cancer patients/chemotherapy (5)*^
  Coronary heart disease patients (30)*+
  Healthy individuals (41)*•
  Hypertension in the elderly (8)*^
  Coronary artery bypass patients (29)*•
  Cancer (152)*
  Senior citizens (25)*•
  Middle-aged women (3)*•^
  Hypertensive patients (11)*•^

C *Page 145*
Cancer
  Quality of life (21)*•
  Pain, anxiety (134)•
  Pain, anxiety post-operatively (57)•
  Anxiety (24)•
  Pain, anixiety post-operatively (151)•
  Pain, nausea, relaxation (22)•
  Pain (158)•+
  Pain, anxiety (4) *•^
  Pain, anxiety (5)*^
  Fatigue (152)*
  Nausea, vomiting, fatigue (23)*•
  Chemotherapy (Blood pressure, Pulse rate, General fatigue, Mood status, Foot fatigue) (5)*^
  Radiotherapy (Fatigue, anxiety, mood) (152)*
  Nausea, vomiting (143)•
  Post-operative pain and anxiety (157)*
  Pain, anxiety, spirituality (140)
  Quality of life (168)*
  Endocrinological and immunological parameter (168)+
Cerebral palsy (49)*+
Cervical spondylosis (116)*+; (50)*+
Cholesterol and triglycerides in the blood
  Hyperlipimia (8)*^
  Hyperlipimia patients (84)*; (86)*+
  Hyperlipimia (85)+
  Menopausal women (12)*^
  Hypertension (58)*
Chronic fatigue syndrome (153)
Chronic obstructive pulmonary disorder (COPD) (149)*•
Circulation (foot) (120)+; (104)
Circulation (Peripheral/diabetes) (6)*^
Colic (138)

Constipation
  Premenstrual syndrome (15)*^
  Students (19)*^
  Women 30-60 (60)
  Elderly (59)*
  Children (Parent/Carer delivered) (61)*
  Children (90)*•
Coronary heart disease (30)*+

D *Page 148*

Deafness (Loss of hearing due to drug toxic effects)(117)
Depression
  Nursing home patients with dementia (31)*•
  Osteoarthritis patients (13)*^
  Pneumoconiosis patients (1)*^
  Elderly women (39)*•+
  Students (19)*^
  Middle-aged women (3)*•^
  Menopausal women (37)*•
  Soldiers (Post traumatic stress syndrome) (132)
  Victims of community violence (Post traumatic stress syndrome) (133)
  Nursing home residents/palliative care (31)*•
  Cancer (140)
Diabetes (Type 2)
  Fasting blood glucose levels (33)*•+
  Fasting blood glucose levels (34)*+
  Blood flow to the feet (35)*
  Pulse, fatigue, mood (7)*^
  Peripheral neuropathy (6)*^
Digestive system (69)*•
Dyspepsia (83)+

E *Page 150*

Edema in pregnancy (148)*•
Encopresis in children (Fecal incontinence / Chronic constipation) (90)*•
Enuresis, Children (7 to 11 years) (52)*•
Enuresis, Children (5 to 10 years) (154)
Enuresis, Children (3-12 years old with history of enuresis for 2-10 years) (126)+
Epilepsy (91)+

F *Page 151*

Falls (Control over for seniors) (25)*•
Fatigue
  Diabetes type 2 (7)*^
  Cancer (24)•; (8)*^; (4)*•^
  Pneumoconiosis (2)*•^
  Premenstrual syndrome (15)*^
  Hospitalized stroke (18)*^
  Elderly women (16)*^

   AIDS (42)*
   Female nurses (9)*^
   Menopausal women (12)*^
Free radicals (51)*+; (50)*+

G *Page 152*
Gout (115)*+

H *Page 152*
Headache (92)
Heart
   Healthy individuals (26)*;
   Healthy individuals (137)
   Coronary heart disease (30)*+
Hemodialysis
  (10)*^; (40)*^; (155)
Hepatitis B (118)+
Hospice (80)•; (136)*•

I *Page 153*
Immune system
   Middle aged women (3)*•^
   Hemodialysis patients (10)*^
   Hemodialysis patients (40)*
Incontinence *See also Enuresis.*
   Middle-aged women (36)*•
   Middle-aged women (17)*^
   Men (109)+
Infertility (84)*; (164)*
Insomnia (See also Sleep)
   Pneumoconiosis (2)*•^
   Premenstrual syndrome (15)*^
   Insomnia (54)
   Insomnia (87)*+
Irritable bowel (55)*•; (56)

K *Page 154*
Kidney function
   Hemodialysis patients (10)*^
   Hemodialysis patients (40)*
   Healthy volunteers (69)*•
Kidney stones (Recovery from lithotrity) (78)*+
Kidney stones (Pain) (74)*

L *Page 155*
Lactation in new mothers (96)*+
Lipoprotein (High density and low density)
   Hyperlipimia patients (84)*
   Hyperlipimia patients (86)*+
   Hypertension in elderly (8)*^
   Hypertension (58)*

   Menopausal women(12)*^
   Hypertension (11)*•^
Lower back pain (93)*; (105)*

M *Page 156*
Menopause (89)*+; (12)*^; (37)*•
Mental health (88)
Mental health (Severe and enduring) (150)
Mental health (Post traumatic stress syndrome) (132); (133)
Mental retardation (95)*+
Middle-aged women (Depression, Perceived stress, Systolic blood pressure, Natural-killer cells and Ig G (antibodies)) (3)*•^
Migraine headache (130); (94)*
Mood
  Diabetes type 2 (7)*^
  Hemodilaysis patients (10)*^
  Hemodilaysis/cancer patients 40)*
  Post-traumatic stress disorder (132)
Multiple sclerosis (98)*; (97)*; (167)
Myopia (119)+

N *Page 157*
Nervous exhaustion (100)
Neurodermatitis (99)*+
Neuropathy (6)*^

O *Page 157*
Osteoarthritis (13)*^; (144)*
Ovulation (164)*
Oxygen saturation (124)+

P *Page 158*
Pain
  AIDS (42)*
  Birthing (48)
  Birthing (47)*
  Cancer (22)•
  Cancer (134)•
  Cancer (151)•
  Cancer (157)*
  Cancer (21)*•
  Cancer (57)•
  Chest pain (73)
  Dementia (patients with) (31)*•
  Diabetes mellitis (6)*^
  Gout (115)*+
  Healthy individuals (88)
  Herniated disc (72)•
  Irritable bowel syndrome (56)
  Kidney stone (74)*

   Knee replacement surgery (141)*
   Lithotrity (78)*+
   Lower back pain (93)*
   Lower back pain (chronic) (105)*
   Miscellaneous pain suffererd (76)+
   Open heart surgery (106)*
   Osteoarthritis (13)*^
   Osteoarthritis (144)*
   Phantom limb syndrome (67)•;
   PMS, Dysmennorhea (15)*^;
   Senior citizens (25)*•
   Sinusitis (77)*
Peptic ulcer (156)*+
Phantom limb pain (67)•
Pneumonia (102)+
Polycystic ovaries (103)
Post operative (Recovery and pain)
   General surgery patients (101)*
   Surgery of cranium or brain (114)+
   Open heart surgery patients (106)*
   Knee replacement (141)*
   Cancer (157)*
   Post abdominal surgery (81)*
   Post gynecological surgery (82)*
   Post prostatectomy surgery (143)*
   Unknown (107)*
Post-partum women
   Women recovering from Cesarean section/Gastrointestinal function (163)*
   Women recovering from Cesarean section / Urinary system (159)*+
   Anxiety, depression (158)*+
   Anxiety, depression, lactation (160)*+
   Triclyceride levels (14)*^
Post traumatic stress syndrome (132); (133)
Premenstrual syndrome (38)*•; (15)*^
Prostate (108)
Pulse rate
   Healthy individuals (41)*•
   Nursing home residents (31)*•
   Cancer chemotherapy patients (42)*
   Healthy individuals (137)
   Senior citizens (28)•
   Coronary heart disease patients (30)*+
   Healthy volunteers (137)
   Hemodialysis (40)*
   Cancer (152)*
   Middle-aged women (3)*•^

R *Page 163*
Respiration (124)+
S *Page 163*
Sinusitis (77)*
Sleep
  Nurses (9)*^
  Insomnia (87)*+
  Insomnia (54)
  Neurodermatitis (99)*+
  Senior citizens (25)*•
  Post traumatic stress syndrome (132)
  Elderly women (39)*•+
  Elderly women (16)*^
  Pneumoconiosis (2)*•^
  Athletes (53)*+
  Cancer (151)•
Stroke (18)*^; (125)+

T *Page 164*
Triglycerides
  Hypertension (11)*•
  Postpartum women (14)*^
  High cholesterol patients (83)+
  Hypertension in the elderly (8)*^
  Menopausal women (12)*^
  Hypertension (58)*

U *Page 165*
Urinary tract infection (112)*+
Urinary tract stones (Lithotrity) (78)+
Urinary tract stones (111)+
Urination
  Men (109)+
  Children (7 to 11 years) (52)*•
  Children (5 to 10 years) (154)
  Children (3-12 years old) (126)+
  Middle-aged women (17)*^
  Middle-aged women (36)*•

W *Page 166*
White blood cell count (low) (121)*+

Chapter Eight: Benchmarks for Dosing and Results   167

Real time as technique is applied
Single session
Daily session (For: two days; three days; one week etc.)
Five times a week
Twice in 24 hours

Two sessions over 4 days
Three times a week
Twice a week
Once a week
Three times a week
Twice a week
Once a week
15 sessions
13 sessions
12 weeks
12 sessions
11 weeks
10 sessions
10 times over 15-30 days
7-10 sessions
6 sessions over 60 days
6 sessions
4-6 sessions
9 sessions over 19 weeks
4 phases for 40 minutes over 8 weeks
8 times
6 weeks
4 or more sessions
19 times over 5 or 6 months

Chapter Nine: Formula for Hand Reflexology, Self-Help Reflexology, Tool Use 177

Chapter Ten: Discussion of Negative Outcomes   182

Chapter Eleven: Control Groups: Impact on Outcomes 198

(See also discussion and summary page 30.)

Bibliography   206

Introduction

Reflexology research shows that systematic patterns of pressure technique application create specific changes in the body and its health. Evidence found in research provides answers about two issues: what results can be obtained through reflexology work and how to get results with reflexology. Consequently, it is now possible to make evidence-based predictions about reflexology and dosing: the amount of reflexology work needed to achieve a specific outcome.

Results from some 168 reflexology studies are reported here. The studies were selected because abstract or full study information included an indication of how much reflexology work lead to reported results. This included information about the frequency (how often) and/or duration (how long) of technique application. They, thus, met the major goals of this work—assessing reflexology research to determine parameters for success (or failure) with reflexology technique application as well as dosing information.

Some of the studies follow the rigorous standard of science: inclusion of treatment and control groups; randomized assignment of participants to treatment or control groups; blinding or double blinding; publication in peer reviewed journals; and listing with PubMed, the National Institute of Health database. Studies are included, however, which are outside of these standards. This has been done to provide information that serves as a starting point for exploring guidelines for reflexology technique application: frequency (how often), duration (how long) and strength of signal (how hard). Such information is important for those who would conduct rigorous scientific research as well as those who seek to apply reflexology as professional practitioners, care givers and/or self-help users.

This work includes discussions as well as tables of information. Discussions include: general factors impacting successful outcomes (page 21), general results of reflexology work (page 32), negative outcomes (page 178) and control group factors (page 193). Tables include information about procedures and outcomes (page 40) and specific dosing and results (pages 117, 126, 133, 138, 163, 173). Included also is the Bibliography of 167 studies.

Chapter One

Factors
Impacting Research and
Successful Outcomes

Key
* Controlled study
• PubMed (National Institute of Health)
^ Published in a peer-reviewed journal (Korea)
+ Published in a peer reviewed journal (China)

Factors Impacting Successful Outcomes and Research

Factors impacting successful outcomes and research include: technique application, interpreting efficacy and control groups.

Technique application: Its role in successful outcomes

Reflexology work impacts the body as sufficient technique application is applied to prompt change. A cumulative conditioning effect is achieved by consideration of technique application and its frequency, duration and intensity (amount of pressure). To explore this premise, we examined more than 160 studies.

Frequency (How often technique is applied)

How much conditioning—what frequency of technique application—is required to create change? Frequency matters. Of the studies with negative outcomes, insufficient frequency of technique application offers a possible explanation for many.

As an example of how frequency of technique application can impact outcomes, consider studies about cholesterol level. No statistically significant difference was shown in two studies: (A) 50 minute sessions twice a week for 4 weeks with hypertensive patients (58)* and (B) twice a week sessions for 6 weeks with menopausal women (12)*^. On the other hand, two studies showed that foot reflexology work "produced remarkable results" if applied daily: (A) 30-40 minutes 5 or 6 times a week with high cholesterol patients (84)*+ and (B) 30-40 minutes a week for 12 days for hyperlipimia patients and (86)*+.

In another example, two studies showed negative outcomes for those with asthma: Reflexology work was applied in 60-minute sessions once a week for 10 weeks (44)*• and (139)*• showing negative outcomes. Yet, reflexology applied 40-50 minutes daily for 2 to 12 weeks demonstrated a disappearance of symptoms (142)*+.

Enuresis is a third example: "… reflexology given as 14 treatment sessions over a period of four months did not result in a significant fall in enuresis nocturna in children aged seven to eleven years old." (52)*• In contrast: "It is reported that "good effect" resulted from foot reflexology treatment of 38 children with enuresis (over a regimen of daily application for 15 days)" (126)+

As a rule, frequency matters yet frequency issues vary from condition to condition and client to client. That is to say, there are successful outcomes with reflexology applied once a week and/ or twice a week, change in cortisol levels, for example. (31)*• (12)*^ (167) It may be that cholesterol, asthma and enuresis require more frequency of reflexology work to achieve a positive outcome. It is premature to state that reflexology is not effective until conflicting research results are clarified with further research taking into account frequency of technique application.

Duration of reflexology session

Discussion of the duration of the reflexology session is limited here as its inclusion is limited in research abstracts and studies. One study, however, serves as an example that demonstrates the limitations of a short duration session for chronic problems. One study found no significant difference in pain following a 15-minute application for sufferers of osteoarthritis. (144)* Also, a one-time fifteen-minute application of reflexology work for edema in pregnancy demonstrated significantly improved wellbeing but not a decrease in the circumference of the ankle (148)*•.

Short but frequent reflexology work has been shown to be effective. 10-minute sessions applied frequently (five days a week for five weeks) produced significant results for hemodialysis patients (10)*^. Results included: improvements in waste product removal, red blood cell level, immune system as well as increases in vigor, mood, uplift, and self-care.

Just as with frequency, an appropriate duration of session varies from condition to condition and client to client. Multiple studies show results achievable with a one-time short amount of reflexology work for: Pain relief (22)• (102)+ (134)• (74)* (45)*• (48) (64) (65)• (66)• (137); Relaxation (64) (65)• (66)• (137) and Anxiety reduction. (41)*• (21)*• (23)*• (134)• Examples of these studies include benefits of a short duration session with cancer patients. A significant decrease in pain relief for cancer patients was found with a 30-minute partner delivered session. (21)*• A 10-minute session with cancer patients "produced a significant and immediate effect on the patients' perceptions of pain, nausea and relaxation." (22)•

Amount of pressure / Intensity

In a sort of Goldilocks effect, too little or too much pressure application can make the difference in successful outcomes. To consider the ramifications of intensity (amount of pressure) in technique application, Chinese researchers conducted a study demonstrating results when techniques of moderate strength were applied in comparison to those of low strength. (124)+ They found "Remarkable and significant results produced by stimulation applied of moderate strength as opposed to low strength: Oxygen saturation rate for moderate strength: 20.50 and for low strength: 17.17; Respiratory rate for moderate strength: 98.73 and for low strength: 97.50."

"The difference between them was remarkable. … if improper strength of stimulation was applied, the following consequences might be induced: (1) If the strength of stimulation is too weak it won't be enough to induce the effective reaction of the body; (2) If the strength of stimulation is too strong, it could induce not only endurable pain, but also low cardiac output … "The researchers also note observations from their clinical experience. The client's sensitivity should be assessed according to sex, age, and 'constitution.'"

While the amount of pressure applied during the reflexology work is not often reported in study results, it should be. This would also help with another aspect of reporting on reflexology research: variations in technique applied by individual reflexologists and individual reflexology methods.

When it comes to protocol and research design for reflexology research, such principles can make differences in outcomes. Questions are raised where possibly too little pressure was applied to produce results. For example, following a gentle pressure reflexology application for 60 minutes to healthy individuals, participants showed no significant difference from the control group in measures of "trait anxiety": cortisol, melatonin or diastolic blood pressure. (41)*• Results did include "Powerful anxiety-reduction effect" with a significant difference in systolic blood pressure and pulse rate.

Once again appropriateness is an issue. The authors of this study (McVicar et. al.) note their long time successful use of a light pressure technique application with cancer patients. If cancer patients rather than healthy individuals had been the participants in the research, would the outcome have been the same? Further research is needed to determine if a more moderate level of pressure would effect "trait" (cortisol and melatonin) anxiety measures for healthy individuals in a single session.

In another example, post surgical recovery studies (81)* (82)* showed foot massage with (presumably) a lighter pressure to produce better results than the application of reflexology technique.

Reflexology method

Reflexology methods vary in their approaches and this may impact outcomes. In one study, a light touch method of reflexology was utilized to test recovery from knee surgery. (141)* Mixed results were obtained. Reflexology methods with cream, oil or lotion technique application form an unknown variable in research. At issue is whether or not: this is in point of fact foot massage; an appropriate level of pressure to obtain reflexological results can be achieved; and, thus, if research results would be different when using a "dry" technique application. Since use of oil, cream or lotion is not reported in studies, its impact on study outcomes is not known. Whether or not these are important issues will become clear with further research. However, the reporting of details in research reporting such as reflexology method, use of oil etc. and amount of pressure is necessary for accuracy of research.

Mode of technique delivery (Foot reflexology, Hand reflexology, Self-help reflexology)

By far, more research has been conducted on reflexology applied to the feet by another (practitioner, individual trained for the study or family member). However, research has demonstrated positive outcomes with the application of hand reflexology and self-help reflexology techniques. Hand reflexology provides the advantage of ease of access while producing results, for example, for those undergoing hemodialysis (10)*^(11)*•^.

Self-help reflexology provides the advantages of patient involvement, the potential for frequency of application and the consideration of money savings. Self-help hand reflexology was found to make a "highly significant difference" and to be "effective in eradicating or reducing pain" for those with phantom limb pain (67)•. Research has been conducted and demonstrated positive outcomes through multiple self-help foot reflexology methods: hands-on techniques (6)*^ (9)*^ (11)*•^(17)*^; electric foot roller (63); standing mat (104); cobblestone path (25)*•; bamboo stepping (158)*+ (166); and massage sandals (120)+.

Application by another is generally believed to be more relaxing. One research study supports this contention. Daily self-help application for six weeks did not show a change in cortisol (3)*•^, a measure of "state" relaxation. As noted above, a significant difference was shown when technique was applied by another once a week for four weeks (31)*• and twice a week for 6 weeks (12)*^ with a difference shown when applied once a week for 6 weeks (167).

Reflex areas (Where technique is applied)

Within reflexology work, application of technique to the appropriate reflex area is of key importance. Central to reflex area selection is an overall premise: technique is applied to a reflex area that mirrors a part(s) of the body involved in creating change in a function. Such change results in improvements such as symptoms and physiologic measures.

One study shows the importance of appropriate work. Reflexology work was applied to the "renal tract zone" of incontinent women 45-minutes a day for three weeks. Reflexology was found to be effective for a lessened day time micturation rate but did not create a difference in 24-hour micturation frequency (36)*•. The issue is raised, does incontinence result from problems with the kidneys or problems with the nervous system's instructions sent from brain to kidneys and, thus, reflexology work to be applied to the corresponding reflex area? Results were achieved, for example, when the cerebral reflex area was included in work with childhood enuresis. (126)+ Had work been applied to the brain stem reflex area in (36)*• would a better result have been achieved?

Does reflexology work applied to a specific reflex area effect the reflected part of the body? Research shows two views. Two studies demonstrated that technique applied to a specific reflex area impacted the related organ. Doppler sonogram measurements before, during and after reflexology technique application to the kidney reflex area showed increased blood flow to the kidneys. (69)*• A similar study found technique application to the intestine reflex area showed increased blood flow to the intestines. (68)*• On the other hand, a study of reflexology work following knee replacement surgery (141)* shows the complexities of working with reflex areas. Recovery was the same for participants receiving reflexology work applied to the knee reflex area of the foot and those receiving reflexology work applied to reflex areas not pertinent to the knee.

Further research will shed light on possible differences between reflexology work that effects a reflected part of the body and reflexology work that ameliorates pain in a reflected part of the body.

The human variable: the client, the reflexologist and the medical practitioner
From the practitioner to the patient to the medical system itself, people make a difference in reflexology and in research. Research and reflexology results are impacted by the illness of the patient, the reflexology method employed by the practitioner, the skill of the practitioner, and bias by the medical personnel involved.

The issue is summed up by Philip Tovey in writing about his research on reflexology work and irritable bowel syndrome (IBS): "For instance, we need to examine the varying impact of individual practitioners and indeed the extent to which the legitimacy held by orthodox practitioners, for instance general practitioners and/or nurses, might impinge on the effectiveness of reflexology. And even with IBS, as noted above, varying the definition and selection of patients may yet yield different outcomes." (55)*•

The illness of the patient is a factor. For those recovering from acute, abdominal gynecological surgery, for example, foot reflexology actually made things worse. (82)* Bringing awareness to the body through reflexology work may not be a good idea when the individual's body is experiencing such an extreme situation. Both long-time reflexologists and Chinese researchers recognize the role of technique applied appropriately to the individual with consideration of frequency, duration and strength.

Skill of the practitioner and bias of medical personnel are difficult if not impossible to gauge. Replication of research would seem to be a remedy. Questions are sometimes raised, however, by things such as reporting of results. An abstract posted at entrezpubmed, for example, obscures positive results obtained in a study of menopausal symptoms. (37)*• (See "Reporting of Results, page 27.")

Questions are also raised when outcomes are contrary to general findings from other studies. For example, research found that reflexology did reduce systolic blood pressure but not anxiety in patients following coronary by-pass surgery (Anxiety) (29)*•. This is contrary to eight studies showing reduction, decrease or significant decrease in anxiety: (Cancer) (134)•; (Healthy individuals) (41)*•; (Cancer) (21)*•; (Cancer) (23)*•; (Coal workers pneumoconosis) (1)*^; (Student nurses) (19)*^; (Palliative care) (80)•. Results could be explained by any one of the human factors: the illness of the patient, the skill of the reflexologist, the type of reflexology utilized or the support of the medical personnel involved. Or, it could be that reflexology is not effective in this instance. The outcome does appear to be an aberration.

Impact of multiple factors

Designing reflexology protocols and research to target specific results requires an examination of all factors: frequency, duration, intensity, delivery systems, reflex areas and the human factors such as health of participants in the study. To impact measures of trait anxiety (cortisol, melatonin or diastolic blood pressure), for example, both amount of pressure and frequency may provide the keys to reaching such a goal. A one-time application with light pressure applied to healthy individuals did not show a change in trait anxiety. "This is an expected result since trait anxiety, unlike state (anxiety as measured by systolic blood pressure and pulse rate), is not a transitory state and any changes in trait anxiety would not be expected in the time-course of this study (one session)." (41)*•

Cultural and historic factors

Results can vary depending on the country where the research was conducted. As noted above, Tovey raises the issue of impact on research due to bias in the medical system. In a similar vein, there is an impact on research varying with societies where reflexology use is a traditional part of the culture and those where it is not. While it is difficult to weigh possible ramifications, it does add interest to a review of research.

To some extent the sheer number of reflexology studies by country makes a statement. More studies are reported in Denmark - fourteen - than the United States - thirteen. Considering the populations of each, the inequity is apparent. The pattern of reflexology in each country makes a statement. In Denmark, surveys have shown that reflexology is the most popular complementary and alternative medical practice with some 25% of the citizens using it regularly. In the US, chiropractics is the most used followed by massage therapy.

Interesting to note also is who conducts the research. In this report, China leads the way in numbers of studies with more than 50 studies followed by Korea with 20 studies. In China, research is conducted by medical doctors and in Korea by nurses. And, the studies reported here are likely to be the tip of the iceberg. Research from China and Korea lacks broader circulation due to language differences and communication gaps. This is demonstrated by a report from Korea. Young-hae Chung, PhD of Dongshin University in Korea notes: "There were 59 master's and doctoral theses and peer reviewed articles on foot reflexology published in Korea from January 1990 to December 2006" (as compared to the 20 Korean studies reported here).

Few studies are reported in Austria and the Netherlands, countries with deeply entrenched reflexology use. It is almost as if there is no need to prove with research something so widely believed and so much a part of the culture. However, in Germany as noted by the Reflexology in Europe Network Web site "It will be clear that reflexology in Germany is only applied on a limited scale and that research is non-existent owing to the particular situation (legal difficulties in preacticing reflexology) in this country." (http://www.reflexeurope.org/countries%20pages/Germany.html)

Numbers of negative studies also make a statement. Some one-third of studies in Denmark result in negative outcomes. By contrast, a report from China reports a 6% "not effective" rate in a review of 8,096 cases and 63 disorders. In Chinese research, reflexology work is commonly applied in a series of ten daily sessions followed by an evaluation. Work proceeds for another ten day cycle if needed to achieve desired goals. There are several ways to consider this pattern. Long time reflexologists nod in agreement. They understand that frequency of technique application is a key component of reflexology work. That there is no time limit to reflexology's application during Chinese research makes good sense. After all how else could you discover how much reflexology work is needed to impact a particular disorder? The issue is, thus, not Will reflexology impact the disorder? but How long will it take? and What will be the efficacy? (how many of the study's participants will be significantly effected, effected or not effected). Such a statement speaks volumes about the entrenchment of reflexology in the Chinese culture.

With experience comes knowledge. The Chinese researchers have demonstrated that with sufficient conditioning through reflexology application, the body can be prompted to behave in a better manner. The change can be so dramatic as to eradicate illness. The Chinese study of urination in men over 55 found that some were "cured" with reflexology "Significantly effective (cure") in 48.68% of all cases." For 44.95% of study participants, reflexology was shown to be "Effective or improvement," thus, offering a way to effectively ameliorate their frequent urination.(109)+

Interpreting Efficacy

See also: Chapter Ten: Discussion of Negative Outcomes, page 182

Can the interpreting or reporting of results obscure the actual outcome? Several studies raise questions about the responsibility of the researcher to fully and fairly disclose results or issues that could skew results.

Reporting of results: Its importance in clarifying outcomes

Can the reporting of results obscure the actual outcome? One study of menopause's physical and psychological symptoms raises such a question. (37)*•

While the reported results may be accurate, they obscured the basic fact: a positive impact on menopause was achieved through reflexology work. Foot reflexology was applied to participants in the treatment group and foot massage to those in the control group. At http//www.entrezpubmed.gov (official US government site), the posted abstract for the study noted: "Foot reflexology was not shown to be more effective than non-specific foot massage in the treatment of psychological symptoms (anxiety and depression) occurring during menopause...."Reflexology could not be shown to be more effective than non-specific foot massage in relieving menopausal symptoms."

In another abstract of the study it is reported:
"Results: Anxiety and depression scores fell in both groups to between 50% and 70% of baseline values, with a clear time effect but no significant difference between treatment and control groups. Similar changes were found for severity of hot flushes and night sweats. "Conclusions: Reflexology could not be shown to be more effective than non-specific foot massage in relieving menopausal symptoms." (http://positivehealth.com/permit/Updates/rudwomen2.htm)

On-line comments form Sandra Goodman note: "It is most unfortunate that the conclusions as written in the above abstract stated that reflexology was not more effective than non-specific foot massage. 99.9% of readers will take this to mean that reflexology was not effective for menopausal symptoms. This is not what really appears to be what happened in this study, which is that foot massage and reflexology both reduced menopausal symptoms of anxiety, depression, hot flushes and night sweats by some 30%-50% of what they were at the outset. The real conclusion of this study is that foot massage is probably not a reliable control procedure for reflexology. (Comment from Sandra Goodman, PhD posted at http://positivehealth.com/permit/Updates/rudwomen2.htm)

The primary researcher and author Jan Williamson acknowledged in on-line comments: "Both groups treatment and control in this study experienced improvements in psychological symptoms during the menopause. Therefore, the study highlights the beneficial effects which can be achieved by therapies which work on the feet. Research into complementary therapies is sparse and even more so into reflexology in particular. Thus, when studies are undertaken, the focus needs to be on the scientific rigour of the study. However this study does show the problem of devising an appropriate placebo control trial of reflexology. Future studies may benefit from the lessons gained here by avoiding attempts at blinding, eliminating the complication of non-specific effects, perhaps by using a waiting group for instance." Jan Williamson (Comment posted at http://positivehealth.com/permit/Updates/rudwomen2.htm)

Quantitative vs. qualitative measures (Patient's view vs. objective measures)
Researcher Helen Poole raises the questions: "Should the patients' view of efficacy be negated because 'objective' measures showed no effect? or the appropriateness of the scientific parameters questioned because they are in conflict with patients notion of efficacy?"

In Poole's research into chronic lower back pain, 243 participants were randomized to one of three groups (reflexology, relaxation or non-intervention (usual care by GP)). Analysis measurements (ANOVA) "...found no significant differences between the groups pre and post treatment on the primary outcome measures of pain. ... There was a main effect of pain reduction, irrespective of group." However, "...interview data revealed that the majority of participants reported treatment led to reduction in pain, increased relaxation and an enhanced ability to cope." ... "The quantitative data suggest that reflexology is ineffective for managing CLBP (Chronic Lower Back

Pain), while the qualitative data suggest otherwise. This incongruence between results raises important questions for the design of research studies into the efficacy of CAMs. Should the patients view of efficacy be negated because 'objective' measures showed no effect? or the appropriateness of the scientific parameters questioned because they are in conflict with patients notion of efficacy? Whatever the verdict it is apparent that studies which consider treatment outcome need to define that outcome in terms that have currency for providers and consumers alike." (105)*

A similar question was raised in research of Chronic Obstructive Pulmonary Disorder (COPD) (149)*•. Patients felt they had benefited from taking part in this study, indicating that there were changes in sleeping patterns, breathing, and the ability to cope with life. There was no evident change in the patients' quality of life when assessed by the quality of life questionnaires. "More research is needed into this areas, since any changes in the quality of life over this short period of time may not have been picked up by the quality of life questionnaires...."

Timing of measurement

Timing of measurements involved in research can raise questions about outcomes.

A question was raised about the negative outcome of a hospice study. (136)*• Reflexology work did not show a greater effect over simple foot massage and did not demonstrate a cumulative effect in anxiety and depression. Dr. Nancy Stephenson has noted that: "Measurements were made prior to the first treatment and within 24 hours of the last treatment. Immediate post measurement was not recorded; the delay may have been the reason the study did not show immediate benefits for decreasing symptoms such as pain and nausea. Patients made positive comments and were relaxed." (Stephenson, Nancy, "Partner delivered reflexology ..." commenting on Ross, C S., Hamilton, J, Macrae, G, Docherty, C, Gould, A, Cornbleet, M A (2002). "A pilot study to evaluate the effect of reflexology on mood and symptom rating of advanced cancer patients," *Palliative Medicine* 16: 544-545)

Baseline measurements

Baseline measurements became a matter of concern for one cross over study.

In a cross over study with multiple sclerosis patients (167), measurements were taken pre-treatment and post-treatment, however, "despite the 4 week break (between one treatment, reflexology and the other, training for progressive muscle relaxation) most outcome measures did not return to pre-treatment levels." Positive effects for both therapies were reported, however, researchers noted "limited evidence of difference between the two treatments, complicated by the ordering effects."

Blinding

How difficult is it to blind reflexology research? And does this impact outcomes? In two studies such questions were raised.

"Subjective scores and bronchial sensitivity to histamine improved on both regimens but no differences were found in the groups receiving active or placebo reflexology. However, a trend in favour of reflexology became significant when a supplementary analysis of symptom diaries was carried out. At the same time a significant pattern compatible with subconscious un-blinding was found. Discussion: We found no evidence that reflexology has a specific effect on asthma beyond a placebo influence." Asthma (139)*•

"In the reflexology group, more (incontinence) patients believed they have received "true" reflexology (88.9 vs. 67.4%, p = 0.012). This reflects the difficulty of blinding in trials of reflexology. Larger scale studies with a better-designed control group and an improved blinding are required to examine if reflexology is effective in improving patients' overall outcome." (36)*•

"However this (menopause) study does show the problem of devising an appropriate placebo control trial of reflexology. Future studies may benefit from the lessons gained here by avoiding attempts at blinding, eliminating the complication of non-specific effects, perhaps by using a waiting group for instance." Jan Williamson (Primary author of study) (37)*• (Comment posted at http://positivehealth.com/permit/Updates/rudwomen2.htm)

Summary of blinded studies
Double-blinded: Asthma (139) *•; Blood pressure (Baroreceptors) (26)*; Diabetes mellitus (Type 2) (34)*+; Intestines (Blood flow / Doppler) (68)*•; Kidneys (Blood flow / Doppler) (69)*•

Single-blinded: Cancer (Quality of life) (151)•; Colic (138); Constipation (61)*; Dementia (31)*•; Diagnosis (146); Edema (148)*•; Incontinence in middle-aged women (36)*•; Irritable bowel syndrome (55)*•; Lower back pain (93)*; Migraine headache (94)*; Ovulation (164)*

Control Groups: Placebo Reflexology, Sham Reflexology and Foot Massage

See also Chapter Eleven: Control Groups: Impact on Outcomes, p. 182

A review of control groups shows "… the problem of devising an appropriate placebo control trial of reflexology." As noted above, one observer states that "The real conclusion of this study is that foot massage is probably not a reliable control procedure for reflexology." This could be especially true for use of the same practitioner to provide both reflexology to the treatment group of a study and then foot massage to the control group of the same study. In four of five such studies, the outcomes were the same for treatment participants (reflexology) and control (foot massage) participants.

Sham reflexology was defined in studies as: technique applied to reflexology areas other than those pertinent to the area of research or technique applied with an attempt not to "hit the points" (apply pressure to appropriate reflex areas).

Use of sham or placebo reflexology as a control
Fourteen reflexology studies were conducted using placebo reflexology or sham reflexology work. In the sham or placebo reflexology an attempt was made not to "hit the points," i.e. apply pressure to appropriate reflexology areas or use a light pressure. Of these fourteen:
• 6 found reflexology work to be "Better than the placebo or sham reflexology work:" Cancer (UK) (151)•, Intestinal function (Austria) (68)*•, Kidney function (Austria) (69)*•, Multiple sclerosis (Israel) (98)*, PMS (US) (38)*•
• 4 found reflexology work to be "Better in some respects, no better in others:" AIDS (Thailand)

(42)*, Knee replacement surgery recovery (UK) (141)*, Edema (Australia) (148)*•, Low back pain (Italy) (93)*
• 1 found "Sham reflexology (with gentle massage) may have a beneficial general effect (but not genuine reflexology), which this study was not designed to detect." (Ovulation) (UK) (164)*
• 1 found reflexology work to be "Same as the placebo reflexology or sham reflexology work" (Positive outcome) Colic (Denmark) (138)
• 2 found reflexology work to be "Same as the placebo reflexology or sham reflexology work" (Negative outcomes) Asthma (Denmark) (139)*•, Asthma (Denmark) (44)*•
• One study utilized Sham TENS and found reflexology work to be "Better than the placebo" Pain threshold and tolerance (UK) (75)

Use of foot massage as a control

Eleven studies were conducted using foot massage as the control group or one of the control groups. Of the eleven:
• 4 found reflexology work to be the same as foot massage: Heart baroreceptors (Healthy subjects) (UK) (26)*; Hypertension patients (Australia) (58)*; Hospice /palliative care (UK) (136)*•; Menopause (UK) (37)*•
• 6 found reflexology work to be "Better in some respects and foot massage better in others:" Constipation in children (Scotland) (61)*, Heart baroreceptor (UK) (26)*, Osteoarthritis (Joint pain) (US) (144)*, Incontinence (Hong Kong) (36)*•, Post surgical recovery (Austria) (81)*, Menopause (UK) (37)*•.
• 1 found foot massage work to be "Better:" Post surgical recovery (Austria) (82)*

In five of the eleven studies, reflexology and foot massage work was provided by the same practitioner. Of these five:
• 4 found reflexology work to be the same as foot massage with positive outcome for both groups: Heart baroreceptors (Healthy subjects) (UK) (26)*; Osteoarthritis (Joint pain) (US) (144)*; Hospice /palliative care (UK) (136)*•; Menopause (UK) (37)*•
• 1 found reflexology work to be the same as foot massage with negative outcome: (Hypertension patients) (Australia) (58)*

The providing of reflexology and foot massage by the same practitioners was an issue recognized by one researcher. As noted by Schoolmeesters: "A limitation was the researcher administering all interventions and questionnaires." (US) (144)*

Chapter Two

What Reflexology Research Demonstrates

Key

* Controlled study
• PubMed (National Institute of Health)
^ Published in a peer-reviewed journal (Korea)
+ Published in a peer reviewed journal (China)

What Reflexology Research Demonstrates

Reflexology research demonstrates the effect of reflexology on a variety of physical and psychological concerns:
• Impact on specific organs
• Amelioration of symptoms
• Creation of a relaxation effect
• Impact on physiological measures
• Improvement in blood flow
• Aids in pain reduction
• Beneficial for post-operative recovery and pain reduction
• Enhancement of medical care
• Adjunct to mental health care
• Complement to cancer care
• Easier birthing / delivery / post-partum recovery

Summary of results

Of the 78 disorders and 168 studies reviewed in this document, research shows an efficacy of 93.3% (11 negative outcomes) by one measure and 80.12% by another (11 negative outcomes and 22 positive-negative outcomes). The positive-negative studies showed at least one positive measure and at least one negative measure or impact as good as results of control group. An example is a study of middle-aged women (3)*•^ found: significant difference following reflexology work in depression, perceived stress, systolic blood pressure, natural-killer cells and Ig G but no significant difference in diastolic blood pressure, pulse or serum cortisol.

Impact on specific organs

Application of reflexology's pressure techniques has specific impact on specific organs. The feet are tied into the whole body due to their role in the body's "fight or flight" mechanism. Just as the body prepares its internal organs to provide the fuel for either eventuality, the feet too play their part, preparing to fight or flee as needed. The sudden adrenaline surge that enables a person to lift a car to free a trapped individual is an example of this reaction. Note that the feet are a part of this action just as they are a part of making our way through each day. Sensing of pressure by the feet makes these roles possible.

Reflex areas in the feet mirror the body's image. Such a method is common within the nervous system, helping to keep track of the location of the body. An image of the body is reflected in five regions of the brain, most notably the homunculus or "little man" in the sensory cortex. Through such reiteration, an on-going flow of information keeps the feet up-to-date about the functioning of other parts of the body. The feet can thus be informed about what kind of response the adrenal gland, for example, can support and then act appropriately in response to moving through the day or a fight or flight demand.

Research using Doppler sonogram and fMRI demonstrates such effect. In one study using Doppler sonogram to measure the impact of the work, it was shown that reflexology work applied to the kidney reflex area of the foot prompted an increase in blood flow to the kidneys (69)*•. Similarly in another Doppler sonogram study, reflexology technique applied to the intestinal reflex area created an increased blood flow to the intestines (68)*•. One fMRI study showed that reflexology technique applied to the reflex area reflecting the right side of the head and brain activated that same area in the brain (127). Another demonstrated that stimulus applied to the eye, shoulder and small intestine reflex areas resulted in activation of the somatosensory area corrsponding to the foot and also the somatosensory areas corresponding to the eye, shoulder and small intestine (visceral and cutaneal of the trunk). (169)

An ECG measured the results of reflexological stimulation (to the heart reflex area) just below the toes of both feet by a mechanical reflexological device (Massage-scroller type) (63). "The effectiveness of reflexology stimulation on the heart rate variability (HRV) signal was measured by three means: correlation dimension analysis (CD), entropy and Poincare plot geometry (SD2 (m s)." "Reflexology being a healing work working on the subtle planes of the human body, we are using subtle tools for investigating the same." Results: The three parameters of cardiac function were compared and in "most of the cases under study due to the effect of reflexological stimulation have changed significantly."

Amelioration of symptoms

The impact of reflexology on disorders is documented in research. The specifics of this impact are as complex as the body itself. First, the application of reflexology's pressure techniques effects the body. Research of its real time and single session application provides such information. Next, think of reflexology work as a conditioning process. Most of the research documented here involves the application of technique over time and illustrates the conditioning process. This documentation consists of patterns of reflexology technique application, their frequency and duration.

Review of the research suggests that reflexology works within a complex body process, one in which the pattern of disorder is integrated into the workings of the body. A variety of the brain's and body's processes are involved thus requiring re-integration of them through a pattern of reflexology technique application appropriate to the disorder.

To more fully consider these ideas, we start by noting examples. Testing has demonstrated that real-time reflexology technique stimulation to a specific reflex area has impact in the reflected part of the body. In addition, research shows that reflexology work applied over time impacts disorders of those body parts.

For example, Doppler sonogram shows blood flow in the kidneys of the urinary system as reflexology work takes place. (69)*• In addition, research shows that reflexology impacts disorders of the urinary system. Impact to the functioning of the kidney was demonstrated when hand reflexology was applied to dialysis patients over time (10 minutes, five days a week for 5 weeks) creating a positive change in three measures of the kidney's functioning (waste product removal, red blood cell level, immune system). (10)*^ Further research demonstrated impact on those with kidney stones - easing pain (74)* and making possible the quicker the excretion of fragmented calculus after lithotrity. (78)+ In a study of reflexology applied to men with prostate problems, 65% reported a reduction in their need to urinate, (67%) reported a better bladder pressure and 80%

reported reduced sexual problems. (109)+ For middle-aged women, reflexology research showed: urinary incontinence reduced, vaginal contraction improved and daily life discomfort reduced. (17)*^ For children, bed wetting was made better as shown by two studies.(154) (126)+

In another example, during the application of reflexology work to the intestinal reflex area of the foot, Doppler sonogram showed increase in blood flow to the intestines. (68)*• Impact of reflexology work on a function of the intestines was demonstrated by three studies of individuals with constipation. For individuals in various ages groups, reflexology work over time ameliorated symptoms: the elderly (reflexology work daily for 10 days) (59)*+, middle-aged women (15 sessions of reflexology work) (60), and children (12 weeks of reflexology work) (61)*.

In a more complex example of a body process, a single session reflexology technique application did not show a change in cortisol (41)*• while a pattern of sessions weekly for 4 weeks did show a change (31)*• as did a pattern of twice a week sessions for six weeks (12)*^ and a pattern of once weekly for six weeks (167). Conclusion: integrative activity is required to create change in the cortisol level, activity created with the application of reflexology over time.

How much conditioning with what frequency is required to create change? Frequency matters. As previously noted, cholesterol level provides an example. Three studies showed that foot reflexology work "produced remarkable results" if applied daily (30-40 minutes 5 or 6 times a week for 20 sessions, for high cholesterol patients (84)*+; 30-40 minutes a week for 12 weeks for hyperlipimia patients and 30-40 minutes daily for 12 days for high cholesterol patients) (85)+. No statistically significant difference was shown for sessions of 50 minute twice a week for 4 weeks. (12)*^

Creation of a relaxation effect

Multiple studies using a variety of measurements show that reflexology relaxes the body. The stimulation of reflexology's pressure techniques creates change in the body's basic level of tension as demonstrated by research using measurement of: brain waves (EEG), blood pressure, systolic blood pressure, diastolic blood pressure, pulse rate, and anxiety. One study of a single session noted that reflexology has a "… powerful anxiety-reduction effect …." (41)*•

Measurement by EEG / Brain Waves

The EEG (electroencephalogram) measures electrical activity of the brain. When we're awake and active, the brain wave pattern created by electrical activity is distinctively different from when we're relaxed or sleeping. In five different studies, EEG (brain waves) measurements were tracked as reflexology work was applied. In three studies, reflexology work was applied to the foot as a whole (64) (66)• (137) and, in two, technique was applied to the part of the hand reflecting the brain, the upper one-third of the thumb (65)• (70). All found that reflexology work created brain waves associated with relaxation, alpha and theta brain waves. One study found that when foot reflexology work began, significant increases were seen immediately in the alpha and theta waves. (64)

Blood pressure was significantly decreased, decreased or lowered for participants in 7 studies
• Significant difference (Coronary heart disease patients) (30)*+; (Hypertensive patients) (11)*•^
• Significantly greater decrease (Nursing home residents) (31)*•

- Decrease (Healthy volunteers) (137); (Elderly with hypertension) (8)*^
- Lowered (Senior citizens) (28)•; (Healthy volunteers) (137)
- No significant difference (Healthy individuals) (26)*

Systolic blood pressure was significantly decreased, decreased or lowered for participants in 9 studies. (Systolic blood pressure is a measure of sympathetic nervous system activity.)
- Significant difference (Healthy volunteers) (41)*•; (Cancer patients/chemotherapy (5)*^; (Cancer chemotherapy patients) (42)*
- Decrease in (Elderly with hypertension) (8)*^
- Lowered significantly (Coronary artery bypass patients) (29)*•; (Coronary heart disease patients) (30)*+
- Significantly lower (Cancer) (Hand reflexology) (152)*
- Statistically significant difference (Self-help reflexology): (Middle-aged women) (3)*•^; (Hypertensive patients) (11)*•^
- "… powerful anxiety-reduction effect (state)" including lowered systolic blood pressure (Healthy individuals) (41)*•

Pulse rate was significantly decreased, decreased or lowered for participants in 8 studies
- Significant difference: (Healthy individuals) (41)*•; (Nursing home residents) (31)*•; (Cancer chemotherapy patients) (42)*
- Decreased: (Healthy individuals / Physiological measures) (137)
- Lowered: (Senior citizens) (28)•; (Coronary heart disease patients) (30)*+; (Healthy volunteers) (137); (Cancer) (Hand reflexology) (152)*
- "… powerful anxiety-reduction effect (state)" including lowered pulse (41)*•

Anxiety was significantly decreased, decreased or lowered for participants in 9 studies:
- Reduced: (Healthy individuals) (41)*•; (Menopausal women) (37)*•
- Significant decrease: (Partner delivered) (Cancer) (21)*•; (Cancer: second and third round of chemotherapy) (23)*•; (Coal workers' pneumoconiosis patients) (1)*^ (Cancer) (134)•
- Decreased: (Student nurses) (19)*^
- Relief from: (Palliative care patients (80)•
- Lower: (Cancer patients following surgery) (157)*
- Significantly lower degree of fatigue, anxiety, and mood state (Hand reflexology) (Cancer & radiotherapy) (152)*

Aid in pain reduction

Pain reduction is a significant result of reflexology work. Twenty-seven studies show positive outcomes for reflexology work ranging from "significant difference in" pain to "reduction in" pain.

Of note is the broad range of individuals whose pain is impacted by reflexology work. Included are individuals of all ages and health states: birthing mothers, menstruating women, phantom limb pain sufferers, lower back pain sufferers, kidney stone patients, senior citizens and individuals with pain resulting from surgery. Such a range speaks of impact on an underlying mechanism at work.

To test such a mechanism, a classic test of pain was conducted. Reflexology work was applied to one group of healthy individuals and Sham TENS to another. (88) The individuals then immersed their hands in ice water. Measurements were taken to judge pain threshold (the time it takes for the subject to find the experience painful) and pain tolerance (the time it takes until the subject can no longer keep his/her hand in the ice water). The reflexology group then received sham TENS before ice immersion and the TENS group received reflexology work. When reflexology work was applied before ice immersion, the results showed a significant change in the individuals' ability to perceive pain. There was a significant increase in pain threshold as well as in pain tolerance. With such findings, researcher Carol Samuels notes the possibility of an over-lying mechanism at work when reflexology work is applied.

Researcher Samuels cites the possibility of the Gate Control Theory (GCT) of pain. According to Wikipedia: "Gate control theory asserts that activation of nerves which do not transmit pain signals, called nonnociceptive fibers, can interfere with signals from pain fibers, thereby inhibiting pain." Stimulating nerves that sense touch, heat, cold and pressure overcomes the action of the pain nerves. As an example, hitting one's elbow activates pain nerves but rubbing the elbow sets off nerves that inhibit the action of the pain nerves.

Applied to reflexology, the idea is, thus, the nerve signals of reflexology's pressure technique application to the feet interferes with pain signals elsewhere in the body. This takes place through the complex interaction that is pain perception as hypothesized by reflexology researcher Dr. Nancy Stephenson. In her study on partner reflexology and cancer patients (21)*•, she notes: "… the current use of reflexology for pain relief is based on the Western neuromatrix theory of pain (Loeser & Melzack, 1999; Melzack, 1999). The theory is an expansion of the Gate Control Theory (GCT) of pain that proposes that pain is a multidimensional experience involving three major psychological dimensions: sensory-discriminative, motivational-affective, and cognitive-evaluative.

"The GCT describes pain as a noxious stimulus that could be increased or decreased by modulations in the gating mechanisms (Melzack & Wall, 1982). The sensory-discriminative dimension of pain is affected mainly by the rapidly conducting spinal system. The motivational-affective system is influenced by activities in the reticular and limbic areas of the brain and the slowly conducting spinal system. The cognitive-evaluative component is in the higher brain center, which evaluates and controls the sensory-discriminative and motivational-affective systems (Melzack & Katz, 1994; Melzack & Wall). The neuromatrix theory proposes that pain is produced by neural patterns in the body-self matrix of the brain and that the three dimensions of pain perception overlap (Melzack, 1999).… Reflexology affects the complex inputs and processing in the neuromatrix of the brain (Stephenson & Dalton, 2003)."

Research shows that reflexology has impact on pain in a variety of situations. As noted, twenty-seven studies show positive outcomes for reflexology work ranging from "reduction in" pain to "significant difference in" pain:

AIDS (42)*; Birthing (47)* (48); Cancer (21)*• (22)• (57)• (134)• (151)•; Chest pain (73); Diabetes mellitus (Peripheral neuropathy) (6)*^; Gout (115)*+; Herniated disc (72)•; Irritable bowel syndrome (56); Kidney stones (74)*; Lithotrity (Recovery from) (78)+; Lower back pain (93)*;

Phantom limb (67) •; PMS/Dysmenorrhea (15)*^; Post operatively (101)* (107)* (106)* (143)* (157)*; Osteoarthritis (13)*^; Senior citizens (25)*• (31)*•; Sinusitis (77)*; and Miscellaneous pain sufferers (76)+

Impact on physiological measures

Research shows that reflexology work influences physiological measures of the body. Measures include and demonstrate positive impact on: alpha amylase, blood pressure, systolic blood pressure, pulse rate, blood uric acid level, carbon dioxide (exhaled), cholesterol, cortisol, Doppler sonogram, ECG, EEG, fMRI, free radicals, hemoglobin, oxygen density, oxygen saturation, serotonin, triclycerides, uric acid and white blood cell count as well as immune system, intestinal, kidney and pancreas function. Such measures document that reflexology has an effect, providing an objective yardstick to measure reflexology's effects and offering evidence of reflexology's potential benefits.

For example, two studies tested reflexology and physiologic measures to show benefits for nursing home residents. Both compared nursing home residents who receiving reflexology work to those who didn't. During one study "Physiologic stress was assessed using blood pressure, heart rate, and salivary measures of cortisol, alpha amyase and DHEA." (31)*• (Cortisol is a hormone and indicator of long-term stress. Alpha amyase is a salivary enzyme sensitive to psycho-social stress.) Results "demonstrated a significantly greater decrease in symptoms of pain, depression and physiologic measures of stress for the residents given reflexology treatment than for those in the control group ... "These clinical findings support the use of reflexology in nursing home residents with mild/moderate dementia."

In a study involving elderly women, results showed that the reflexology group had better quality of sleep, less depression and higher levels of serotonin. (39)*•+ (Among other things, serotonin influences psychological functions such as anxiety mechanisms and the regulation of mood, thoughts, aggression, appetite, sex drive and the sleep/wake cycle.) "Conclusion: It's necessary to give foot reflexion massage as a successful nursing intervention to elderly who undergo a change in sleep, and suffer from a depression disorder due to a deterioration in sleep."

Alpha amylase
Statistically significant reduction (Dementia / Nursing home residents) (31)*•

Blood pressure, systolic blood pressure and pulse rate are lowered.
See "Creation of a Relaxation Effect," pages 35-36.

Blood uric acid level
Normalized (Gout) (115)*+

Carbon dioxide (exhaled)
Increased 9% Carbon dioxide density exhaled from nose (Healthy volunteers) (137)

Cholesterol
• Remarkable reduction (High cholesterol patients) (83)+

- Remarkable reduction (Hyperlipimia patients) (84)*
- Marked statistical difference and reduction (High cholesterol patients) (85)+
- Not significantly decreased (total cholesterol level, HDL and LDL cholesterol (Hypertension in the elderly) (8)*^

Cortisol
- Significantly greater decrease (Dementia / Nursing home residents) (31)*•
- Statistically significant differences (Menopausal women) (12)*^
- Difference (Multiple sclerosis patients) (167)
- No significant difference (Post surgical breast cancer) (168)*
- No significant difference (Healthy volunteers) (41)*•
- No significant difference (Middle-aged women)(3)*•^ (Self Foot Reflexology)

Doppler sonogram
- Improvement in blood flow rate, time, and acceleration in lower limbs (Diabetes) (35)*
- Increase in real time blood flow (Intestines) (68)*•
- Effective in changing real time blood flow (Kidney) (69)*•

ECG (Electrocardiogram) (Measurement of heart's activity)
- Improved remarkably (Coronary heart disease patients) (30)*+
- Relaxation indicated real time (Healthy volunteers) (137)
- Change real time in T-waves / Disappearance of angina symptoms (Angina patient) (62)+
- Changed significantly real time (Electric foot massager) (Self foot reflexology) (63)

EEG (Measurement of brain waves)
- Significant increases in one or more patterns: Significant increase in alpha amplitude, theta amplitude,% alpha synchrony and% theta synchrony (Healthy volunteers) (64)

Increase in relaxation waves:
- Increase in alpha frequencies (relaxation waves) in the brain waves (Healthy volunteers) (66)•
- Increase in alpha waves that remained following reflexology work (Healthy volunteers) (137)
- "Brings the brain-mind mechanism to a lower dimensional chaos indicating a state of 'order out of disorder'" (Healthy volunteers) (65)•
- "Results showed that there was a clear differences in characteristics of EEG signals with and without reflexology. Results signal relaxation effect of reflexology." (Healthy volunteers) (70)

fMRI
- Reflexology stimulus applied to lateral inner big toe (left foot) activated reflected region of the brain, the right temporal lobe (127)
- Visual cerebral cortex not activated but reflex area stimulation matched same results as when acupoint stimulated in stroke patients with vision deficits (128)
- Reflexology and acupuncture stimuli resulted in activation in the same area of the brain, the insula demonstrating that both at the point (adrenal gland / K1 used for psychological asthma for both) probably regulate emotional and pain effects. The strongest activation in the brain for pressure applied to the adrenal gland reflex area was the insula with functions of homeostasis, pain, emotions) (129)

• Stimualtion to the eye, shoulder and small intestine reflex areas resulted in activation of the somatosenory areas corresponding to the foot as well as those corresponding to the eye, shoulder and small intestine (visceral and cutaneal/trunk) (169)

Free radicals
• Significant difference SOD (super-oxide dismutase), GHtal (antioxidation activities), MDA (malynol) (Cervical spondylosis) (50)*+
• No difference from control group (SOD: increase; GP: increase; GHtal, MDA: decrease) (Sham reflexology: not applied to symptom appropriate reflex areas) (Healthy individuals/various illness) (51)*+

Hemoglobin
• Increase in hemoglobin (Hemodialysis) (10)*^

Human growth hormone
• No effect (Post surgical breast cancer) (168)*

Immune system
• Increase in lymphocyte subsets; CD32, CD33, CD34; "However, no significant differences between (experimental and control) groups were found for: CD4 increased significantly; NK (Natural killer) cells decreased significantly and CD 8 decreased (Hemodialysis patients) (10)*^
• BT, Pulse Rate and Blood Pressure were decreased significantly on the 1st times, but not 5th times; Hb (hemoglobin) levels significantly increased; Emotional responses, vigor and mood scores were significantly increased; B cell and CD19 were increased significantly; Suppressor T cell and NK (Natural killer) cell showed significant decrease after the program, but no significant differences between the groups. (Hemodialysis patients) (40)*
• Statistically significant difference in (Natural-killer cells and Ig G antibodies) (Middle-aged women)(3)*•^ (Self foot reflexology)

Intestinal function
Increase in real time blood flow rate measured before, during and after work (35)*

Kidney function
Effective in changing Real time blood flow rate measured before, during and after work (68)*•
Significant difference:
• BT, pulse rate and blood pressure were decreased significantly on the 1st times, but not 5th times; Hb (hemoglobin) levels significantly increased (Hemodialysis and cancer patients) (40)*
• Increase in Hb (hemoglobin); Decrease in BUN (blood urea nitrogen) and Cr. (creatinine) (Hemodialysis patients) (10)*^

Melatonin
No significant difference from control group (Healthy volunteers) (41)*•

Oxygen density
Real time: Before: 95-97%; during, increase to 97% (Healthy volunteers) (137)

Oxygen saturation

Remarkable and significant results produced by stimulation applied of moderate strength as opposed to low strength. (124)+

Pancreas function

• Greatly reduced: fasting blood glucose levels; platelet aggregation; length and wet weight of the thrombus; senility symptom scores; serum lipid peroxide (LPO) (Diabetics) (33)*•+
• Marked improvement. effective rate for 67% in: senility, thrombocyte aggregation rates (TAR), the length and wet weights of thrombosis in vitro, and the serum oxidative lipids (Diabetics) (34)*+
• Blood flow rate in feet measured before, during and after work (Diabetes) (35)*

Prolactin

• No effect (Post surgical breast cancer) (168)*

Serotonin

Higher serotonin levels than control group (Elderly women) (39)*•+

Respiratory rate

Respiratory rate lowered (Senior citizens) (28)•

Triglycerides

• Decrease in (Hypertension) (11)*•^; (Postpartum women) (14)*^
• Strong effect (High cholesterol patients) (83)+
• Significantly decreased Hypertension in the elderly (8)*^
• No change (Menopausal women) (12)*^; (Hypertension) (58)*

Uric acid

Blood uric acid normalized (Gout) (115)*+

White blood cell count

White blood cell count improved (Leukopenia) (121)*+

Improvement in blood flow

Improvement in blood flow is one of multiple mechanisms of action at work in reflexology technique application. Research shows that reflexology work applied to a reflex area reflecting a body part prompts an improved blood flow to that body part: kidneys (69)*•, intestines (68)*•, and the brain (fMRI) (127) (128) (129) (169). Research also shows improved blood flow to the feet. (35)*

Beneficial for post-operative recovery and pain reduction

Research shows reflexology to be beneficial following surgery. It aids in recovery and pain reduction as well as lessening the use of post operative analgesics. Negative results from three studies show the further need for tailoring reflexology work to this special circumstance.

Results from research following surgery found:
• Reflexology enhances urination, stimulates bowel movements and so aids recovery. Patients who received reflexology also showed a much less need for medication than patients in the control group (107)*
• This study showed a decrease of the quantity of pain killers in the foot reflexology group to less than 25% - 35% in comparison with control group. (General surgery) (101)*
• Post-operative pain and anxiety among gastric and liver cancer patients recovering from surgery was reduced. (157)*
• Research showed that the mean of unpleasant symptoms score (pain) in the group receiving pre-operative information combined with foot reflexology and aromatherapy was the lowest among three groups. The mean of unpleasant symptoms score in the group receiving preoperative information combined with foot reflexology and aromatherapy was the lowest. (106)*
• "Posttest mean score on pain of an experimental group was significantly lower; Posttest mean score of frequency pain medication taking was significantly lower than of a control group" (Post prostatectomy surgery) (143)*
• For women recovering from Cesarean section, there was a significant difference in time to first defecation for reflexology group. (163)*
• For women recovering from Cesarean section, there was a significantly difference with a shorter voiding time for reflexology group. (159)*+
• "There was no significant difference in any of the three groups (for release from hospital or long term pain killer use), with the exception of morphine consumption in the early postoperative period (48 hours after surgery). Patients receiving real or placebo reflexology treatment used significantly less morphine than the control group." (Knee replacement surgery) (141)*
• The foot reflexology group was more able to void without problems and the indwelling catheter removed earlier. The foot massage control group showed significant results in the subjective measures of well-being, pain and sleep. (Abdominal surgery) (81)*
• Reflexology is not recommended for patients recovering from gynecological surgery. It has various effects, some negative including occasionally trigger abdominal pain. The foot massage control group found the experience more relaxing and positive (Gynecological surgery) (82)*

Enhancement of medical care

Cancer patients, phantom limb pain sufferers, hemodialysis patients, diabetic individuals, neuropathy patients, and many more ill individuals are among those whose need for help exceeds that available through medical practices. For these individuals and others, research has demonstrated that reflexology use enhances medical care to help where medicine can't.

Cancer patients

Research shows that reflexology works: (A) Eases the side effects of chemotherapy, nausea, vomiting and fatigue (4)*•^ (24)•; (B) Reduces anxiety and pain (22)• (134)• (23)*• (57) and depression (140)(3)*•^; and (C) provides a means for family members to add their support (21)*•.

Phantom limb pain sufferers

The sensation that pain exists in a removed limb is known as phantom limb pain. Research shows that reflexology work alleviates and, at times, eliminate phantom limb pain. (67) •

Hemodialysis patients

Patients undergo hemodialysis to replace the functions of failed and failing kidneys. Research shows that reflexology work helps these individuals: Improves the kidney's functions with changes in physiologic measures: an increase in red blood cells (to combat anemia concerns), increase in lymphocytes (to help fight infection), and enhances disposal of waste products. (10)*^ (40)*

Diabetic individuals

Diabetes is characterized by the inability to produce or utilize insulin. For some, there is an unpredictable variation in glucose tolerance, brittle diabetes, that results in difficulty treating it with an appropriate level of medication. Research shows that reflexology work reduces physiologic measures for diabetics and is an effective treatment for type II diabetes mellitus. (33)*•+

Neuropathy patients

Neuropathy patients suffer from nerve degeneration leading to loss of sensation and potentially and, potentially loss of limbs due to poor circulation as gangrene can set in. Diabetics are prone to neuropathy. Research shows improvement in blood flow rate, time and acceleration within the feet following reflexology work. (6)*^ Bead mat walking also showed an increase in blood flow to the feet. (104)

Adjunct to mental health care

Reflexology programs and research show that reflexology aids the mentally ill, providing needed benefits unique to reflexology work. Mental health workers report that reflexology work furnishes many advantages including facilitating communication and allowing for the client to be "touched during treatment in a safe non-intrusive / abusive manner." (88)

Aggressive and anti-social children

Reflexology work with children and young people showed "a reduction in aggression, stress and anxiety and an improvement in focus, concentration, self esteem, listening skills and confidence." Reflexology provided a "specific partial treatments aimed at calming down the children and young people so that their behavior becomes less challenging within the classroom and generally, making the mainstream more accessible." (135)

Autism

Improvements are noted in work with autistic children. (Lamont)

Emotional support

A study followed "30-minute reflexology sessions for eight weeks. The findings included: physical improvements, emotional improvements, self-esteem and confidence, motivation, touch, increase in relaxation levels, being heard and taken seriously, concentration improvements." (88)

Mentally ill (severe and enduring)

A study examined the use of reflexology with individuals "at the severe and enduring end of the mental illness spectrum" (schizophrenia and obsessive-compulsive disorder). "… reflexology was accepted by the clients in terms of their interest, attendance and tolerance of touch. … "The researcher observed that clients who arrived for the session displaying stress, or in one case expressing paranoid ideas, appeared to relax and were calmer by the end of the session It was apparent that clients felt able to talk about a wide range of topics before, during and after the reflexology session. Talking was not the focus of the session and it seemed as if this allowed talking to take place" (150)

Post traumatic stress syndrome

One study found that victims of community violence in Northern Ireland experienced a significant improvement in psychological health and levels of depression over time. (133) Research with Israeli soldiers demonstrated temporary relief from symptoms including anger, depression and muscle tension as well as improved sleep patterns, levels of concentration and a lift in overall mood. Researchers found that improvements lasted three days and suggested sessions two or three times a week to improve their results with once a week sessions. (132) (132a)

Depression

Multiple studies show an improvement in mood or lessening of depression:
• Nursing home patients with dementia: Significantly greater decrease (31)*•
• Osteoarthritis: Significant improvement (13)*^
• Pneumoconiosis patients: Significant decrease (1)*^
• Elderly women: Less depression disorder (39)*•+
• Middle-aged women: Statistically significant difference (Self help foot reflexology)(3)*•^
• Menopausal women: "… reduced menopausal symptoms of anxiety, depression, hot flushes and night sweats by some 30%-50% of what they were at the outset." (37)*•
• Post traumatic stress syndrome: Temporary relief from symptoms including anger, depression and muscle tension; Improved sleep patterns, levels of concentration and a lift in overall mood (Israel) (132)
• Post traumatic stress syndrome: Significant improvements in psychological health and levels of depression over time (Northern Ireland) (133)
• Cancer patients: Lowered levels of depression, anxiety, spirituality; Increased levels of emotional quality of life and total quality of life (140)

Anxiety

Anxiety was significantly decreased, decreased or lowered for participants in 9 studies:
• Reduced: (Healthy individuals) (41)*•; (Menopausal women) (37)*•
• Significant decrease: (Partner delivered) (Cancer) (21)*•; (Cancer: second and third round of chemotherapy) (23)*•; (Coal workers' pneumoconiosis patients)(1)*^; (Cancer) (134)•
• Decreased: (Student nurses) (19)*^
• Relief from: (Palliative care patients (80)•
• Lower: (Cancer patients following surgery) (157)*
• Significantly lower degree of fatigue, anxiety, and mood state (Hand reflexology) (Cancer & radiotherapy) (152)*

Complement to cancer care

Thirteen studies from seven countries (US, Italy, Japan, China, Switzerland, Korea, United Kingdom) target cancer care and show the benefits of reflexology work.

- Anxiety: Decrease in self-reported anxiety (23)*•
- Chemotherapy: Decrease in nausea, vomiting, fatigue (4)*•^
- Chemotherapy: Significant difference in: diastolic blood pressure, pulse rate, general fatigue, mood status, foot fatigue (5)*^
- Depression, anxiety, quality of life: Lowered levels of depression, anxiety, spirituality; Increased levels of emotional quality of life and total quality of life (140)
- Fatigue: Effective for alleviating fatigue (24)•
- Hospice: Patients identified relaxation, relief from tension, feelings of comfort and improved well-being (80)•
- Nausea, vomiting: Bamboo stepping group had a significant impact on nausea and vomiting with an overall efficiency of 90.83% (158)*+
- Pain: Positive immediate effect in pain reduction (57)•
- Pain management, anxiety: Significant decrease in pain and anxiety (134)•
- Pain, nausea, relaxation: Significant and immediate effect on patients' perceptions of pain, nausea and relaxation (22)•
- Pain and anxiety: Significant decrease in pain intensity and anxiety (21)*•
- Post-operative pain and anxiety: "less pain and anxiety over time; "intervention group received significantly less opioid analgesics than the control group" (157)*
- Quality of life: Improved quality of life (151)•
- Radiation therapy: Significantly lower degree of fatigue, anxiety and mood state (157)

Easier birthing / delivery

Reflexology work during pregnancy or delivery creates easier birthing / delivery.
- Analgesia: Less used (45)*•
- Duration of labor: Reduced (46)
- Duration of labor, analgesia: Reduced duration; Effective rate of analgesia 94.4% (47)*
- Labor pains, retention of placenta: 90% effective rate as pain killer; 11 of 14 with retention of placenta avoided operation (48)
- 70% of women diagnosed with primary inertia during labor made progress when treated with reflexology (165)*

Chinese researchers have found reflexology to be beneficial for women throughout the child-bearing experience from conception to post-partum issues:
- Infertility (84)*
- Postpartum Women (158)*+
- Postpartum Women (Anxiety and depression) (160)*+
- Post partum (Urinary system) (159)*+
- Post-partum women recovering from Cesarean section (Gastrointestinal function)(163)*

Research shows that reflexology benefits newborn infants as well. For premature infants (162)*+, those who received reflexology showed "Significant differences in sleep duration and total sleep time as well as better 7-day and 30-day weight gain" in contrast to infants in the Control Group (breast feeding and premature infant care practices).

Chapter Three

Procedures and Outcomes for 169 Studies and 78 Disorders / Physical Conditions

Key
* Controlled study
• PubMed (National Institute of Health)
^ Published in a peer-reviewed journal (Korea)
+ Published in a peer reviewed journal (China)

Procedures and Outcomes

Research	Method	Results: Significant Difference	Results: Other Effects
Subject of Research (Reference number)	**Method** • # of participants • Type of reflexology • Type of study • Length & duration of work	**Results: Significant difference** (Scores changed significantly in the experimental group but not in the control group or changed significantly from pre-reflexology to post reflexology)	**Results: Other Effects**
Aggressive, anti-social behavior in children / Mainstreaming (135)	• Unknown number • Children with emotional and behavioral difficulties • Foot reflexology • 30 minutes • Weekly for 8 to 15 weeks	• Goal of calming down the children and young people so that their behavior becomes less challenging within the classroom and generally, making the mainstream more accessible • Evaluation shows a reduction in aggression, stress and anxiety and an improvement in focus, concentration, self esteem, listening skills and confidence.	
AIDS (42)*	• 28 hospitalized AIDS patients • Foot reflexology • Cross over design • 30 minutes, 2 reflexology and 2 mimic / sham sessions over 4 days	• Significant difference: less pain and fatigue	No significant difference on a 1-item numeric pain intensity scale

Research	Method	Results: Significant Difference	Results: Other Effects
Anxiety, salivary cortisol and melatonin (41)*•	• 30 healthy volunteers • Foot reflexology using "gentle" pressure, 60 minutes • Control group • Cross-over design with 3 days between • Pre-test /post-test at critical times	• "Powerful anxiety-reduction effect" Significant difference in state anxiety (temporary condition) as measured by: • Systolic blood pressure: Significant difference • Pulse rate: Significant difference	No significant difference in trait anxiety (long standing quality) measured by: • Diastolic blood pressure: No significant difference • Cortisol and melatonin: no significant difference
Arthritis (43)+	• 42 individuals with acromioclavicular (shoulder) arthritis • 30 minutes per day for 15 days	• 8 were "cured" • 20 were "distinctly effective" • 14 cases were "improved"	
Asthma (44)*•	• 30 individuals with bronchial asthma • Control group: Care by General Practitioner • 60 minutes per week for 10 weeks		Reflexology and control groups both showed: • Decrease in consumption of beta-2-agonists and increase in peak-flow levels
Asthma (142)*)	• 45 children (ages 1 to 7) with infantile bronchial asthma • Control group • 40-50 minutes daily for 2 to 12 weeks	• Disappearance of symptoms	

Appetite *See Cancer (Quality of life) (151)•; Hospice (136)*; Athletes (153)*+ ; Postpartum women (159)*+*

Research	Method	Results: Significant Difference	Results: Other Effects
Asthma (139)*•	• 40 individuals with bronchial asthma • Control group (placebo reflexology where the specific reflexology areas were not pressed) • Double-blinded • 45 minute, once a week for 10 weeks		"Objective lung function tests did not change. Subjective scores and bronchial sensitivity to histamine improved on both regimens but no differences were found in the groups. A trend in favour of reflexology became significant when a supplementary analysis of symptom diaries was carried out. At the same time a significant pattern compatible with subconscious un-blinding was found. Discussion: We found no evidence that reflexology has a specific effect on asthma beyond a placebo influence."
Birthing (Labor outcomes) (45)*•	• 150 women • Control group of 100 • Some received 4 or more sessions	Reflexology group experienced: • less analgesia used • more forceps deliveries	No difference • onset of labour • duration of labour
Birthing (Relieving labor pains / Birth process) (47)*	• 213 women • Control group of 105 women • Reflexology provided during labor	Reflexology group experienced: • average birth process of 2.48 ± 1.48 hours • effective rate (analgesia) was 94.4%	Control group experienced: • average birth process of 3.32 ± 1.19 hours
Birthing (Relieving labor pains) (48)	• 68 women • Reflexology provided during delivery	• 90% effective rate as a pain killer during delivery • 11 of 14 with retention of placenta avoided operation	

Research	Method	Results: Significant Difference	Results: Other Effects
Birthing (Labor outcomes) (46)	• 37 pregnant women • 10 sessions from 20 weeks to term	Reflexology group experienced: • Average first stage was 5 hours, second stage 16 minutes, and third stage 7 minutes • Compared to textbook figures of 16 to 24 hours' first stage, and, 1 to 2 hour's second stage • Normal Deliveries 89.0% • Inductions 5.4% • Forceps 2.7% • Selective Cesarean Section 2.7% • Emergency Cesarean Section 5.4% • Immunological stress 8.1%	
Birthing (Primary inertia) (165)*	• 99 pregnant women with diagnosed primary inertia during labour • Foot reflexology: two sessions each of 30 minutes conducted by one of two midwives • Single-blinded • Controlled (general supportive care for the same amount of time) • Assessment of dilatation of the cervix was carried out before and after treatment by midwife blinded to group	• When treated with reflexology, 70% of women diagnosed with primary inertia during labour made progress • When offered extra supportive midwifery care, 38% of women actually made progress in labor • All women would have been offered "unpleasant and painful oxytocin augmentation under usual care."	

Research	Method	Results: Significant Difference	Results: Other Effects
Birthing (Recovering gastointestinal function after Cesarean) (163)*+	• 194 women following routine Cesarean section • Foot reflexology (108 women: 3 consecutive days) • Control group (86 women): conventional care	• Significant differences in first time defecation and recovery of gastrointestinal function with	
Blood pressure, pain, control over falls in senior citizens (25)*•	• 48 senior citizens • Foot reflexology mat walking • Pretest/posttest • Control group • 3 / week for 45 minutes over 8 weeks (included 10 minute warm-up of foot reflexology or foot roller use; 5 minute cool down of foot reflexology or foot roller use	• Reductions in diastolic blood pressure • Greatly improved perceptions of control over falls • Significantly reduced daytime sleepiness and pain • Increased psychosocial well-being • Considerable improvements in ability to perform "activities of daily living" • Statistically significant change indicating reduced systolic blood pressure pre-to-post change for the reflexology group only.	
Blood pressure: (Baroreceptor reflex sensitivity, blood pressure and sinus arrhythmia) (26)*	• 24 individuals: • 10 Foot reflexology group • 10 Control / Foot massage group • 4 Control group • Blinded • Pre-test/post-test	• Frequency of sinus arrhythmia after reflexology and foot massage increased by 43.9% and 34.1% respectively • All but Control group showed significantly greater reductions in baroreceptor reflex sensitivity	• No significant difference in blood pressure after intervention

Research	Method	Results: Significant Difference	Results: Other Effects
Blood pressure: Healthy individuals (Anxiety, salivary cortisol and melatonin) (41)*•	• 30 healthy volunteers • Foot reflexology using "gentle" pressure • Control group / Experimental group • Cross-over design: 3 days interval • Pre-test / post-test taken at critical times • 60 minutes	• Systolic blood pressure: Significant difference • Pulse rate: Significant difference	• Diastolic blood pressure: No significant difference • Cortisol and melatonin: no significant difference
Blood pressure: (Coronary heart disease) (30)*+	• 125 patients • Foot reflexology • Control (Pharmacotherapy) group • Pre-test/post-test • 30-40 days of treatment	• Blood pressure/heart rate: reflexotherapy group (before): +185/80 / 86-74 and (after): +160/75 / 72-70 • Blood pressure/heart rate: pharmacotherapy group (before): +180/80 / 78-72 and (after): +160/80 / 76-70 • ECG: reflexotherapy group (before): slight change in T-wave and (after): improved remarkably ECG; • ECG: pharmacotherapy group (before): change in ST-T wave and (after): certain improvement	
Blood pressure: (Depression, Stress Responses and Immune Functions of Middle Aged Women) (3)*•^	• 46 middle-aged women • Self help foot reflexology • Pre-test/post-test • Daily for 6 weeks	• Significant difference in depression, perceived stress, systolic blood pressure, natural-killer cells and Ig G	• No significant difference in diastolic blood pressure, pulse or serum cortisol

Research	Method	Results: Significant Difference	Results: Other Effects
Blood pressure: (Efficacy of Reflexology as a Palliative Treatment in Nursing Home Residents with Dementia) (31)*•	• 80 patients • Foot reflexology • Control group • Pre-test/post-test • 1 / week for 4 weeks, 30 minutes each	• Significantly greater decrease in: blood pressure, heart rate, and salivary measures of cortisol, alpha amyase and DHEA • Significantly greater decrease in pain and depression	
Blood pressure (Hypertension) 11*•^	• 34 • Foot reflexology • Control group • Foot reflexology 2 / week for 6 weeks; Self foot reflexology 2 / week for 4 weeks	Decrease in: • Systolic blood pressure • Triglyceride level Improved: • Life satisfaction	No significant decrease in: • Diastolic blood pressure • High density lipoprotein • Low density lipoprotein
Blood pressure (Hypertension in the elderly) (8)*^	• 34 elderly • Control group • 2 / week for 6 weeks	Decrease in: • Systolic blood pressure • Diastolic blood pressure • Fatigue	No significant decrease in: • Serum levels • High density lipoprotein • Low density lipoprotein
Blood pressure: (Pulse rate, respiratory rate, blood pressure for senior citizens) (28)•	• 20 individuals: • Foot reflexology • Pre-test/Post-test • 1 session	• Pulse rate, respiratory rate and blood pressure were lowered • Average biofeedback and temperature were higher post-test • Provided good circulation, relaxation and comfort	
Blood pressure: (Coronary Artery Bypass Graft (Anxiety)) (29)*•	• 9 patients • Foot reflexology • Control group • Pre-test / Post-test • 30 minutes / 5 days	• Systolic blood pressure lowered significantly	• Anxiety scores were not lower for patients in the control group on all measures • No significant changes were observed for other unknown variables

Research	Method	Results: Significant Difference	Results: Other Effects
Blood pressure (Hypertension) (58)*	• 108 hypertension patients • Foot reflexology 50 minute 2 / week for 4 weeks • Control group: 30-minute light foot massage session without pressure on specific reflexology areas twice a week for four weeks		No statistically significant difference between treatment groups post-intervention. for: • Blood pressure • LDL cholesterol • Triglyceride levels.
Cancer & chemotherapy (5)*^	• 11 patients • Foot reflexology • Pretest/posttest • *Not available*	Significant difference in: • Systolic blood pressure • Diastolic blood pressure • Pulse rate • General fatigue • Mood status • Foot fatigue	
Cancer & chemotherapy (4)*•^	• 34 breast cancer patients • Foot reflexology • Control group • 4 phases for 40 minutes over 8 weeks	Decrease in: • Nausea • Vomiting • Fatigue	
Cancer & chemotherapy (Nausea and vomiting) (158) *+	• 240 cancer patients undergoing chemotherapy • Bamboo stepping (120 patients) three times daily for 20 to 30 minutes unknown number of days • Control group (120 patients)	Bamboo stepping group showed significant impact on nausea and vomiting: • 75 cases (62.50%), effective • 34 cases (28.33%) and the overall efficiency of 90.83%	

Research	Method	Results: Significant Difference	Results: Other Effects
Cancer & radiotherapy (152)*	• 29 cancer patients • Hand reflexology, applied to both hands for ten minutes each time, five times during five days • Control group	Significantly lower: • The degree of fatigue, anxiety, and mood state as measured by questionnaire • Lower systolic blood pressure and pulse rate in the experimental group	• Diastolic blood pressure in the experimental group were not significantly lower than that of the control group
Cancer (Psycho-neuroimmunological response) (168)*	• 183 women, post-surgical breast cancer • Reflexology • Indian head massage group • SIS (self-initiated support) • Randomised • 8 weekly sessions starting six weeks post surgically • Measurements taken at 4 and 10 weeks after cessation of sessions	• Reflexology group: "fewer B lympho-cytes than those receiving SIS (self-initiated support) alone" • Quality of life (QOL): Reflexology was better than massage at Trial Outcome index and Mood Rating Scale Relaxation with no significant difference. • Both groups had statistically significant but modest difference on QOL compared to SIS	• Neither group "had statistically significant effects on any endocrinological and immunological parameters thought to be relevant to an anti-tumour response." (lymphocyte subsets, cytokine production, and hormones, prolactin, cortisol, growth hormone)
Cancer Pain and nausea (22)•	• 87 patients • Foot reflexology • 10 minutes	"… significant and immediate effect on the patients' perceptions of pain, nausea and relaxation"	"no statistically significant effect at 3 hours after intervention or at 24 hours after intervention"
Cancer Pain and anxiety (21)*•	• 86 patients • Partner delivered foot reflexology • Control group (read a book of their choice to their partner) • Both groups: 30 minutes three times a week, minimum of four weeks	Significant decrease in pain intensity and anxiety	

Research	Method	Results: Significant Difference	Results: Other Effects
Cancer (Pain management / Pain and anxiety) (134)•	• 23 breast or lung cancer in an inpatient oncology unit • Foot reflexology • Crossover design • 30 minutes of reflexology one day / 30 minutes of rest on another	• For breast cancer patients, a significant decrease in pain, as measured by the descriptive words of the Short Form-McGill Pain Questionnaire (SF-MPQ); (M=?0.41, SD = 0.71, p =.048) • Significant decrease in anxiety, as measured by the VAS for anxiety, for both breast-cancer patients (n = 13, M =?17.38, \SD = 21.29, p = 0.01) and lung-cancer patients (n = 10, M=?21.6, SD = 25.49, p =.02)	
Cancer Anxiety (second and third round of chemotherapy) (23)*•	• 30 Patients • Control group • Foot reflexology • Pre-test/Post-test/ 24 hours after • 1 session	Decrease of 7.9 points on the subjects' self-reports of anxiety (measured by the Spielberger State-Trait Anxiety Inventory) in the treatment group and of 0.8 points in the control group	
Cancer Fatigue (advanced cancer) (24)•	• 20 patients • Footsoak (3 minutes warm water containing lavender essential oil) • Reflexology / Aromatherapy (with jojoba oil containing lavender for 10 minutes) 8 times	Effective for alleviating fatigue in terminally ill cancer patients	

Research	Method	Results: Significant Difference	Results: Other Effects
Cancer (Pain) (57)•	• 36 Inpatients of metastic cancer • Foot reflexology, 10 minute session, two times 24 hours apart • Pre-test / Post intervention / 3 hours after / 24 hours after	• Positive immediate effect in pain reduction • "…pain scores were lowered by 2.4 points on a 0-10 pain scale in the treatment group compared to the control group immediately post intervention (n = 36, F [1,31] = 9.08, p < 0.01)"	• No statistically significant effect 3 hours after • No statistically significant effect 24 hours after
Cancer (Quality of life) (151)•	• 12 patients • Foot reflexology, 40 minutes • Control group: Placebo reflexology (gentle foot massage that did not stimulate reflexology points) • Blinded for participants • Placebo and reflexology groups received three 40 minute sessions, every other day over a five-day period.	• 33% of the placebo group benefited from an improvement in quality of life compared to 100% of the reflexology group. 100% benefited from an improvement in quality of life: appearance, appetite, breathing, communication (doctors), communication (family), communication (nurses), concentration, constipation, diarrhoea, fear of future, isolation, micturition, mobility, mood, nausea, pain, sleep and tiredness.	

Research	Method	Results: Significant Difference	Results: Other Effects
Cancer (Post-operative pain and anxiety among cancer patients) (157)*	• 61 patients • Foot reflexology applied on days 2, 3, 4 after surgery for 20 minutes in addition usual pain management • Control group: usual pain management	• "… less pain (P <.05) and anxiety (P <.05) over time were reported by the intervention group compared with the control group" • "intervention group received significantly less opioid analgesics than the control group (P <.05)"	
Cancer (140)	• Guided imagery (healing images set to music), and/or • Reflexology (10-minute massage of each hand or foot)., and/or • Reminiscence therapy • 8 weeks	• Lowered levels of depression, anxiety, spirituality; • Increased levels of emotional quality of life and total quality of life	
Cerebral palsy (Growth rates) (49)*+	• 16 children (3 months to 3 years) • Control group • Daily for 30 days	Reflexology group experienced: • Increase in growth quotient of 30-35 in those 3 to 9 months old and 10-15 with those from 1.5 to 3 years	Control group experienced: • Increase in growth quotient was 10-16 for 3-9 months and 9-15 for 1.5 to 3 years
Cervical spondylosis (Degeneration of cervical vertebrae or pad between vertebrae) (116)*+	• Cervical spondylosis patients • 84 (hand reflexology &tui-na group) • 44 (control group) • 20-30 minute session daily for 7 days (Course 1; every other day for 7 sessions (Course 2) to 14 sessions (Course 3)	Treatment group: • Clinical "cure" rate, 49% • Remarkably effective or effective within Courses 1 and 2, 93% Control group: • Clinical "cure" rate, 27% • Remarkably effective or effective within Courses 1 and 2, 49%	

Research	Method	Results: Significant Difference	Results: Other Effects
Cervical spondylosis (122)+	• 45 cases symptoms: dizziness, headache, nausea, unstable steps, sweating • Foot reflexology & Vertebral nerve block therapy (injection of drugs at C5-C6 level of vertebrae) • Daily, 30-40 minutes	• Clinically "cured:" 34 (76%) cases, disappearance of symptoms and return to work • Effective: 9 (20%) cases, symptoms relieved and return to work • No effect: 2 cases (4%)	
Cervical spondylosis (Free radicals) (50)*+	• 80 individuals with cervical spondylosis • Foot reflexology • Control group of 28 (neck traction, 20 minutes, once a day) • 30-40 min. for 12 days	Significant difference: • Superoxide dismutase (SOD) • GHtal antioxidation activities • Malonyl (MDA) content No significant difference between the control (92% effectiveness) and treatment (98.1% effectiveness) groups for clinical effectiveness • Clinical "cure" rate was higher in the treatment group (48.1%) than the control group (28.95%)	
Cholesterol (Hypertension in the elderly) (8)*^	• 34 elderly • Control group • 2/week for 6 weeks	Decrease in: • Systolic blood pressure • Diastolic blood pressure • Fatigue	No significant decrease in: • Serum levels • High density lipoprotein (HDL) • Low density lipoprotein (LDL)

Research	Method	Results: Significant Difference	Results: Other Effects
Cholesterol and triglycerides in the blood (Hyperlipimia)(84)*	• 186 cases • (A) Foot reflexology: 30-40 minute session five or six times a week for 20 sessions • (B) Walking, running or step aerobics 4 to 5 times per week • (C) Ion-introduction therapy (30 minutes per day) • (D) Pharmacology (the drug lipunthyl)	• Groups A, C and D showed remarkable reduction in cholesterol. • Group A and D had strong effect on triglyceride.	
Cholesterol and monoglyceride (Hyperlipimia)(85)+	• 72 cases • Foot reflexology • Control group • Daily for 12 days (except Sunday)	• Reflexo-therapy group showed an improvement of symptoms (headache, insomnia, palpitation or poor memory) of 78% as opposed to 32% for the second group. • Marked statistical difference and reduction in cholesterol and monoglyceride	
Cholesterol (Menopausal women) (12)*^	• 40 • Foot reflexology • Control group • Twice per week for 6 weeks	Statistically significant differences: • Climacteric symptoms (Menopause) • Fatigue • Total cholesterol • Cortisol	No significant difference in: • High density lipoprotein (HDL) • Low density lipoprotein (LDL) • Triglyceride

Research	Method	Results: Significant Difference	Results: Other Effects
Cholesterol (Hypertension) (58)*	• 128 hypertension patients randomly assigned to treatment or control group • Foot reflexology 50 minute twice a week for 4 weeks • Control group: 30-minute light foot massage session without pressure on specific reflexology areas twice a week for 4 weeks		"There was no statistically significant difference between treatment groups post-intervention." No statistically significant difference between treatment groups post-intervention. for: • Blood pressure, • Low density lipoprotein (LDL) cholesterol • Triglyceride levels.
Chronic fatigue syndrome (153)	• 50 patients • Foot reflexology • Daily for 10 days, 30 minutes • Unknown number of 10 day treatment series	Symptoms: dizziness, insomnia, fatigue weakness, muscle pain, palpitation, forgetful, poor diet, movements, sexual dysfunction • Recovered 35 cases (70%): Symptoms completely disappeared, resumed normal work • Improved in 15 cases (30%): Significantly reduced the symptoms, resumed normal work. • Total efficiency of 100%.	

Research	Method	Results: Significant Difference	Results: Other Effects
Chronic obstructive pulmonary disease (COPD) (149)*•	• 20 patients • Foot reflexology, 50 minutes once a week for 4 weeks • Control group	• Reflexology group: short term relaxation that did not continue until the next treatment • Patients felt they had benefited from taking part in this study, indicating that there were changes in sleeping patterns, breathing, and the ability to cope with life. "All of these are qualitative results and would need to have further quantitative results and further qualitative analysis (if possible) before an association with the reflexology can be accurately drawn."	There was no evident change in the patients' quality of life when assessed by the quality of life questionnaires. "More research is needed into this areas, since any changes in the quality of life over this short period of time may not have been picked up by the quality of life questionnaires."
Circulation (Foot) (120)+	• 17 individuals • Massage sandals • Foot blood circulation measured by laser tissue scanning equipment • Pre test / Post test	The pre and post test of foot blood flow ratio was 1:2.087 indicating an increase in foot blood flow. Increase in blood flow was also observed on the screen of the equipment.	
Circulation (Peripheral blood circulation) (Diabetes mellitus (type 2) (6)*^	• 76 (ages 40-79) • Self foot reflexology • Control • 6 weeks • Self-help	Good effect: • Improving peripheral neuropathy (especially tingling and pain) • Improving ability to sense 10-g monofilament	Not effective: • Improving peripheral circulation

Research	Method	Results: Significant Difference	Results: Other Effects
Circulation (Foot), Temperature, Galvanic skin response (104)	• 2 healthy individuals • Stepping on wooden bead mat • 5 minutes	• Speed of blood circulation: average "before" measurement 12.5 centimeters per second / "after" measurement 29.0 cm. per second • Temperature of foot improved with more even distribution over the foot • Galvanic skin response showed improvement in form of fewer deviations from the mean before the stimulus	
Colic (138)	• 63 infants who cried for more than 90 minutes over 24 hours • Groups: Reflexology, Non-effective reflexology, Control • Two weeks • Single-blinded	• 33 of 63 infants reduced crying to less than 90 minutes /13 of them were "cured" (crying for less than or equal to 30 minutes). • The infants who did not benefit "had a significantly better outcome… "than the observation group."	
Constipation (Elderly and healthy volunteers)(59)*+	• 40 residents senior facility • Control group (Healthy volunteers) • Daily for 10 days	Reflexology group: the interval between taking the carbon tablet and first black stool for the constipation group changed from an average of 45 hours to an average of 34 hours. The interval until last black stool changed from 77 hours to 51.5 hours. The healthy volunteers experienced improved bowel function as well.	

Research	Method	Results: Significant Difference	Results: Other Effects
Constipation (Middle-aged women) (60)	• 20 women (30-60 years old) • 15 sessions	Average bowel movement for the women was 4.1 days prior to the study and 1.8 days after. 50% reported a normal stool consistency after the study in comparison to none before.	
Constipation (Children) (61)*	• 184 children • Foot reflexology • 2 Control groups (foot massage, standard care) • Taught to and applied by parents or carers • 12 weeks • Single-blinded	"Significant differences between Reflexology and Control groups in bowel frequency (p,0.05) and total constipation symptom score at 12 weeks"	"…there was a significant difference between reflexology and massage for total constipation symptom score (p,0.05) but not for bowel frequency (p = 0.25
Coronary heart disease (30)*+	• 125 patients • Foot reflexology • Control (Pharmacotherapy) group • Pre-test/post-test • 30-40 days of treatment	• Blood pressure/heart rate: reflexotherapy group (before): +185/80 / 86-74 and (after): +160/75 / 72-70 • Blood pressure/heart rate: pharmacotherapy group (before): +180/80 / 78-72 and (after): +160/80 / 76-70 • ECG: reflexotherapy group (before): slight change in T-wave and (after): improved remarkably ECG; • ECG: pharmacotherapy group (before): change in ST-T wave and (after): certain improvement	

Research	Method	Results: Significant Difference	Results: Other Effects
Deafness (Drug toxic effects) (117)+	• 5 patients • Foot reflexology • Daily for 14-28 days for 40 minutes	Significantly effective: Treatment stopped once the patient could hear a speaking voice from a certain distance.	
Dementia (Efficacy of Reflexology as a Palliative Treatment in Nursing Home Residents with Dementia) (31)*•	• 80 patients • Foot reflexology • Control group • Pre-test/post-test • 1 / week for 4 weeks, 30 minutes each / 120 minutes • Trained data collectors blind to subject group assignment	• Significantly greater decrease in physiological measures of stress: blood pressure, heart rate, and salivary measures of cortisol, alpha amyase and DHEA • Significantly greater decrease in pain and depression	
Diabetes mellitus (Type 2) (6)*^ (Peripheral blood circulation, Peripheral neuropathy)	• 76 (ages 40-79) • Self foot reflexology • Control • 6 weeks	Good effect: • Improving peripheral neuropathy (especially tingling and pain) • Improving ability to sense 10-g monofilament	Not effective: • Improving peripheral circulation
Diabetes mellitus (Type 2) (33)*•+	• 32 • Foot reflexology • Control • 30 days	Greatly reduced: • fasting blood glucose levels • platelet aggregation • length and wet weight of the thrombus • senility symptom scores • serum lipid peroxide (LPO)	
Diabetes mellitus (Type 2) (35)*	• 20 diabetic /15 healthy individuals • Foot reflexology • Doppler sonagraphic pre-test/ Post-test • 1 session	Improvement in blood flow rate, time and acceleration within the feet	

Research	Method	Results: Significant Difference	Results: Other Effects
Diabetes mellitus (Type 2) (34)*+	• 22 • Foot reflexology • Control • Daily for 30 days • Double blind	Marked improvement. effective rate for 67% in: senility, thrombocyte aggregation rates (TAR), the length and wet weights of thrombosis in vitro, and the serum oxidative lipids	Control group: No significant change 20% effective rate
Diabetes mellitus (Noninsulin dependent) (7)*^	• 42 (ages 40 to 70) • Foot reflexology • Control group • 30 minutes, 3/ week	Improvement in: • Pulse rate • General fatigue • Foot fatigue • Mood	No decrease of blood sugar levels
Diagnosis (145)•	• 76 patients examined by 3 reflexologists • Each patient and the therapist graded problems related to 13 different parts of the body.		The statistical agreement may be better than pure chance, but is too low to be of any clinical significance
Diagnosis (146)	• Three reflexologists chose six medical conditions which could be detected most easily and reliably. • Eighteen adults with one or two of these conditions were examined by two reflexologists, blinded to the patients' condition(s)		Despite certain limitations to the data provided by this study, the results do not suggest that reflexology are a valid method of diagnosis

Research	Method	Results: Significant Difference	Results: Other Effects
Diagnosis (147)	• 80 patients examined twice by two reflexologists		The reflexology method has the ability to diagnose (reliable and valid) at a systematic level only, and this is applicable only to those body systems that represent organs and regions with an exact anatomic location.
Doppler sonogram (Kidney) (69)*•	• 32 Healthy men and women • Control group • Foot reflexology • Double blinded • Measured before, during and after reflexology work	• Systolic peak velocity and end diastolic peak velocity was measured in cm/s, and the resistive index a parameter of the vascular resistance • Decrease of flow resistance in the renal vessels and an increase of renal blood flow. These findings support the hypothesis that organ-associate foot reflexology is effective in changing renal blood flow during therapy	
Doppler sonogram (Intestines)(68)*•	• 32 Healthy men and women • Control group • Foot reflexology • Double blinded • Measured before, during and after reflexology work	• Increase in the blood flow in the superior mesenteric artery and the subordinate vascular system (the blood flow velocity, the peak systolic and the end diastolic velocities)	

Research	Method	Results: Significant Difference	Results: Other Effects
Doppler (Circulation in Diabetes mellitus (Type 2)) (35)*	• 20 Diabetic /15 healthy individuals • Foot reflexology • Doppler sonagraphic Pre-test/Post-test • 1 session	Improvement in blood flow rate, time and acceleration	
Dyspepsia (83)+	• 230 Dyspepsia patients • Foot reflexology • Control group (drug therapy) • Once or twice a day for two weeks	• Very effective (98 or 74.2%) • Effective (30 or 22.7%) • Failure (4 or 0.3%)	
ECG (71)	• 3 Individuals • Electrical stimulation to simulate reflexology work	"Under reflexology, the complexity (quantified by dimension) of the dynamics was lower compared to without reflexologic stimulations with a general drop as degree of stimulation increased. ... "This implies that dynamics become less complex and the horizon of predictability increase during reflexology."	
ECG (Heart rate variability) (63)	• 20 individuals • Electric foot roller • Real time for 20 minutes • Heart rate variability signal was measured by three means: correlation dimension analysis, entropy and Poincare plot geometry	• Most of the cases under study have changed significantly due to the effect of reflexological stimulation • Measurement by ECG showed a moderate improvement of cardiac function of the heart's activity	

Research	Method	Results: Significant Difference	Results: Other Effects
ECG: (Coronary heart disease) (30)*+	• 125 patients • Foot reflexology • Control (Pharma-cotherapy) group • Pre-test/post-test • Daily, 30-40 days of treatment	• ECG: reflexotherapy group (before): slight change in T-wave and (after): improved remarkably ECG • ECG: pharmacotherapy group (before): change in ST-T wave and (after): certain improvement • Blood pressure/heart rate: reflexotherapy group (before): +185/ 80 / 86-74 and (after): +160/75 / 72-70 • Blood pressure/heart rate: pharmacotherapy group (before): +180/ 80 / 78-72 and (after): +160/80 / 76-70	
ECG (Angina) (62)+	• Case study • Foot reflexology • Real time • 10 days for 50 minutes	• Applied during an active onset of angina and observed with EKG showed disappearance of symptoms and a change to T-waves in V1.3 elevated from depressed T-waves and T-waves in V5 inverted upright from an inversion of T-waves • 10-day course of daily 50 minute, nocturnal attacks of premature beats were relieved though premature beats still occurred occasionally	

Research	Method	Results: Significant Difference	Results: Other Effects
Edema (Pregnancy (148)*•	• 55 women • "Relaxing" reflexology techniques • Specific "lymphatic" reflexology technique • Control: Period of rest • 15 minutes • Single blinded	"A 'perceived wellbeing' score revealed the lymphatic technique group significantly increased their wellbeing the most, followed closely by relaxing techniques and then the control rest group. • From the women's viewpoint, lymphatic reflexology was the preferred therapy with significant increase in symptom relief."	• There was no statistically significant difference in the circumference measurements between the three groups; however, the lymphatic technique reflexology group mean circumference measurements were all decreased. • (All groups) had a non-significant oedema-relieving effect.
EEG (64)	• 10 individuals and 4 who did not produce usable data • Foot reflexology session • Real time	• 10 of 11 showed significant increases, over the course of the session, in one or more of the following measures: alpha amplitude, theta amplitude,% alpha synchrony and% theta synchrony • "Additionally, and perhaps more importantly, there was a substantial drop in these measures immediately following the baseline period when the hands-on portion of the session began."	

Research	Method	Results: Significant Difference	Results: Other Effects
EEG (65)•	• 8 individuals • "Reflexological stimulation of the brain reflex area of the hand" (pressure applied to upper half of thumb) • Real time	"We conclude that reflexological stimulation, from the signals and systems point of view bring the brain-mind mechanism to a lower dimensional chaos indicating a state of 'order out of disorder'... "We expected this, as reflexology claims to de-stress and bring relaxation to the brain."	
EEG (66)•	• 30 subjects • "Foot reflexologic stimulation" • Control group (Classical music followed by rock music) • Both compared to resting state	"… number of parallel functional processes active in the brain is less and the brain goes to a more relaxed state. This gives rise to the increase in alpha frequencies in the brain waves."	
EEG (70)	• 2 Subjects • "Electrical stimulation to simulate reflexology work was applied to the brain reflex 'point' on the thumbs"	• "Results showed that there was a clear differences in characteristics of EEG signals with and without reflexology. Results signal relaxation effect of reflexology: Under reflexology stimulation frequency components are below 30Hz. Normal EEG signal (50-60Hz)"	

Research	Method	Results: Significant Difference	Results: Other Effects
EEG (Physiological measure) (137)	• 5 volunteers • 10 minute foot reflexology session tested • 20 minute reflexology session tested	• Heart rate, blood pressure: decreased • Carbon dioxide density exhaled from nose: increased 9% • EEG (increase in alpha wave) and ECG (fall in interval ratio) both indicate increase in relaxation • Abdominal respiration rate declined slightly	
Encopresis (Fecal incontinence / Chronic constipation) (90)*•	• 50 children • Foot reflexology • 30 minutes once a week for 6 weeks	• Incidence of soiling decreased and bowel motions increased • Soiling before: 78% once daily; 16% once to three times a week; 6% none in a seven day period • Soiling after: 20% once daily; 30% once to three times a week; 48% none in a seven day period; 2% (missing data) • Bowel motions before: 36% none in a seven day period; 46% 1-4 motions per week; 18% daily • Bowel motions after: 2% none in a seven day period; 72% more than 1-4 motions per week; 24% daily	

Research	Method	Results: Significant Difference	Results: Other Effects
Enuresis (52)*•	• Children (7 to 11 years) • Control group • 14 sessions over 4 months		No effect
Enuresis (154)	• 20 Children (5 to 10 years) • 30-minute treatments, twice weekly for four weeks (with a minimum of 2 days between treatments), followed by weekly treatments for seven weeks.	"A decrease in the night time amount of urine was reported by 43.8% of the parents, and 23.5% moved from the category of 'soaking wet' to 'a little wet'"	
Enuresis (126)+	• Children (3-12 years old with history of enuresis for 2-10 years) One course of treatment = 15 sessions daily Reflex areas: cerebral, spine, lumbar vertebrae, solar plexus, adrenal gland, ureter tubes	Good effect	
Epilepsy (91)+	• 9 cases • Daily for 2 to 3 months	• Effective for 8 of the 9 cases • One individual remained off medication 4 years after treatments	

Research	Method	Results: Significant Difference	Results: Other Effects
fMRI (128) (Vision)	• 10 healthy volunteers • Apply reflexology technique applied to left foot, eye reflex area at bases of second and third toes to see if this would activate the visual cerebral cortex	Activation of brain: • Left frontal lobe (Strongest activation) (Polysensory / Premotor area/Language related movement (writing)) • Cerebellum (Conduct impulses to cerebral cortex / Posture, balance, coordination of movements) • Left insula	Visual cerebral cortex not activated but reflex area stimulation matched results when acupoint stimulated in stroke patients with vision deficits: activation of frontal lobe and insula
fMRI (129) (Adrenal gland reflex area stimulation compared to acupuncture K1 (comparable acupoint))	• 14 healthy males • pressure applied to adrenal gland reflex area • electrical stimulation of K1 acupoint • Hypothesis: reflex area stimulation would activate the same brain region as acupuncture stimulation; selected area of left foot (adrenal gland reflex area and K1) is related to emotional disorder and pain (adrenal gland and K1 are utilized to work with psychological asthma)	The activation by both in the insula demonstrated that reflexology or acupuncture stimuli at the point (adrenal gland / K1) probably regulate emotional and pain effects. Activation of brain (reflex area): • Insula (Homeostasis, pain, emotions) (Strongest activation) • Homunculus of the cerebral cortex (Sensory) • Parietal lobe (Premotor) Activation of brain (acupoint): • Homunculus (Sensory) • Insula (Homeostasis, pain, emotions) • Working memory	

Research	Method	Results: Significant Difference	Results: Other Effects
fMRI (127) (Temporal lobe activation)	• 10 healthy subjects • Apply reflexology stimulation to inner lateral corner of the left great toe to see if this would activate the part of the brain reflected by this reflex area, the right temporal lobe	Activation of brain: • Temporal lobe (strongest) (Sensory pathways and/or memory, auditory or language functions) • Cerebellum (Motor-sensory pathway) • Right claustrum (Secondary somatosensory cortex) • Right anterior central gyrus (Tactile stimulation and movement of toe during work)	
fMRI (Eye, shoulder, small intestine reflex areas) (169)	• 25 healthy subjects • Reflexology stimulation applied by stick to eye, shoulder and stomach reflex areas	Resulted in activation in the brain of "somatosensory areas corresponding to the foot but also the somatosensory areas corresponding to the eye, shoulder and small intestine (both visceral and cutaneous trunk) or neighboring body parts"	
Fatigue and sleep (Nurses) (9)*^	• 40 nurses • Self foot reflexology • Control group • 40 minutes, 2/week for 4 weeks	• Score of fatigue decreased • Score of sleep states increased in the study	
Fatigue (Athletes (53)*+	• 12 athletes • Foot reflexology • Control group • Daily for 15 days	Better: • Qualities of sleep • Appetite • Quicker recovery from fatigue and muscle soreness	

Research	Method	Results: Significant Difference	Results: Other Effects
Free radicals (Cervical spondylosis) (50)*+	• 80 individuals with cervical spondylosis • Foot reflexology • Control group of 28 • 30-40 min. for 12 days	Significant difference in: • Superoxide dismutase (SOD) • GHtal antioxidation activities • Malonyl (MDA) content	
Free radicals (51)*+	• 56 individuals with various illness • Control group of 20 healthy medical students • Both groups: 30-40 min. for 10 days Reflexology group: "symptomatic reflexes and related reflexes" were worked for a longer time and with more strength.	Both groups: • Increase blood superoxide dismutase (SOD) and glutathione peroxidase (GP) • GHtal antioxidation activities • Decrease malonyl (MDA) content	
Gout (115)*+	• 15 cases • Foot reflexology • 30 minutes • 7 - 10 sessions	Relieved 100% of symptoms within 7 to 10 sessions: Swollen joint, pain, difficulty in walking, blood uric acid normalized	
Headaches (92)	• 220 headache patients	• Three months after series of reflexology treatments: 81% of patients confirmed that reflexology had either "cured" (16%) or helped (65%) their symptoms. 19% were able to completely dispense with the medications they were taking before the study.	

Research	Method	Results: Significant Difference	Results: Other Effects

See also Migraine headache

Research	Method	Results: Significant Difference	Results: Other Effects
Hemodialysis (10)*^	• 43 hemodialysis patients • Hand reflexology • Control group • 10 minutes, five / week for five weeks	• Increase in Hb (hemoglobin) • Decrease in BUN (blood urea nitrogen) and Cr. (creatinine) • Increase in lymphocyte subsets; CD32, CD33, CD34 • Increases in vigor, mood, uplift, self-care	• CD4 increased significantly; NK (Natural killer) cells decreased significantly and CD8 decreased "However, no significant differences between (experimental and control) groups were found."
Hemodialysis and Cancer: physiological, emotional responses and immunity responses of the patients with chronic illness (40)*^	• 54 hemodialysis and cancer patients • Hand reflexology • Control group • 10 minutes, five times over 3 days	• BT decreased significantly on both of the 1st and the 5th application. • Pulse rate and Blood pressure were decreased significantly on the 1st times, but not 5th times. • Hb (hemoglobin) levels significantly increased • Emotional responses, vigor and mood scores were significantly increased. • B cell and CD19 were increased significantly	• Suppressor T cell and NK (Natural killer) cell showed significant decrease after the program, but no significant differences between the groups.
Hemodialysis (HD) and Cramping (Common to HD patients) (155)	• 5 chronic hemodialysis patients • Self foot reflexology • 10 minutes daily (66% compliance rate)	• Cramp incidences were decreased from 7.8 to 2.8 during HD and from 10.6 to 5.4 at "interdialytic period after implementation of reflexology" • Reflexology in 11 of the 19 incidences of cramp during HD, six incidences (54.5%) relieved, five (45.5%) were not	

Research	Method	Results: Significant Difference	Results: Other Effects
Hepatitis B (118)+	• 4 patients • Foot reflexology • Daily for 40 days	"Cured" of Hepatitis virus: • HBsAg decreased and disappeared	
Herniated disc/ lumbro-sacral (Pain) (72)•	• 40 individuals • Foot reflexology • 3 sessions in 1 week	• 62.5% reported a reduction in pain	
Herpes zoster (114)+	• 100 individuals • Foot reflexology • Every other day	• Significantly effective ("cured") after third session	
Hospice (136)*•	• 26 patients with advanced cancer • Foot reflexology • Control group: Foot massage provided by reflexologists • Weekly for 6 weeks	"Measurements were made prior to the first treatment and within 24 hours of the last treatment. Immediate post measurement was not recorded; the delay may have been the reason the study did not show immediate benefits for decreasing symptoms such as pain and nausea. Patients made positive comments and were relaxed." (21)*•	The study did not show a greater effect of reflexology over simple foot massage and did not demonstrate a cumulative effect in anxiety and depression.
Hospice (80)•	• 34 patients receiving palliative care at a specialist palliative care unit • 4-6 sessions of reflexology • Foot reflexology	Patients identified: • Relaxation • Relief from tension and anxiety • Feelings of comfort and improved well-being	

Research	Method	Results: Significant Difference	Results: Other Effects
Hyperlipimia (Cholesterol and triglycerides in the blood)(84)*	• 186 cases • (A) Foot reflexology: 30-40 minute session 5 or 6 times a week for 20 sessions • (B) Walking, running or step aerobics 4 to 5 times per week • (C) Ion-introduction therapy (30 minutes per day) • (D) Pharmacology (the drug lipunthyl	Groups A, C and D showed remarkable reduction in cholesterol. Group A and D had strong effect on triglyceride.	
Hyperlipimia (Cholesterol and monoglyceride)(85)+	• 72 cases • Foot reflexology (41 individuals) • Control group (20 minute session with a forehead pillow application of iodineiontophoresis) • Daily for 12 days (except Sunday)	• The reflexo-therapy group showed an improvement of symptoms of 78% as opposed to 32% for the second group with headache, insomnia, palpitation or poor memory. • Marked statistical difference and reduction in cholesterol and monoglyceride	
Hypertension in the elderly (8)*^	• 34 elderly • Control group • 2/week for 6 weeks	Decrease in: • Systolic blood pressure • Diastolic blood pressure • Fatigue	No significant decrease: • Serum levels • High density lipoprotein (HDL) • Low density lipoprotein (LDL)

Research	Method	Results: Significant Difference	Results: Other Effects
Hypertension (11)*•^	• 34 • Foot reflexology • Control group • Foot reflexology 2 / week for 6 weeks; Self foot reflexology 2 / week for 4 weeks	Decrease in: • Systolic blood pressure • Triglyceride level Improved: • Life satisfaction	No significant decrease in: • Diastolic blood pressure • High density lipoprotein • Low density lipoprotein
Hypertension (58)*	• 128 hypertension patients randomly assigned to treatment or control group • Foot reflexology 50 minute twice a week for 4 weeks; • Control group: 30-minute light foot massage session without pressure on specific reflexology areas twice a week for 4 weeks		"There was no statistically significant difference between treatment groups post-intervention." No statistically significant difference between treatment groups post-intervention. for: • blood pressure, • LDL cholesterol • triglyceride levels.
Immune System (Hemodialysis) 10*^	• 43 hemodialysis patients • Hand reflexology • Control group • Hand reflexology • 10 minutes, five / week for five weeks/ 250 minutes	• Increase in Hb (hemoglobin) • Decrease in BUN (blood urea nitrogen) and Cr. (creatinine) • Increase in lymphocyte subsets; CD32, CD33, CD34 • NK (Natural killer) cells decreased significantly • CD4 increased significantly • Increases in vigor, mood, uplift, self-care	• CD8 decreased "However, no significant differences between (experimental and control) groups were found."

Research	Method	Results: Significant Difference	Results: Other Effects
Immune System (Depression, Stress Responses and Immune Functions of Middle Aged Women) (3)*•^	• 46 middle-aged women • Self Foot reflexology • Pre-test/post-test • Daily for 6 weeks	• Significant difference in depression, perceived stress, systolic blood pressure, Natural Killer (NK) cells and Ig G	• No significant difference in diastolic blood pressure, pulse or serum cortisol
Incontinence in middle-aged women (17)*^	• 39 middle-aged women • Self foot reflexology • Control group • 30 minutes 3/week for 4 weeks	• Urinary incontinence reduced • Vaginal contraction improved • Daily life discomfort reduced	
Incontinence in middle-aged women (36)*•	• 109 middle-aged women • Foot reflexology • Control group (foot massage) • 45-minutes daily for 3 weeks • Single blinded	• Significant change in the number of daytime frequency in the reflexology group	• 24-hour micturition frequency in both groups, but the change was not statistically significant
Infertility (84)*	• 4 women who tried to become pregnant • Foot reflexology • Course of treatment: 30-40 minute session daily for 10 days	• One woman became pregnant after 6 courses of treatment • Two after seven courses • One after nine course	
Infertility / Ovulation (164)*	• 48 women • Foot reflexology group (26 women) • Sham reflexology with gentle massage (22 women) • Single-blinded • 8 sessions over 10 weeks		"The rate of ovulation during true reflexology was 11 out of 26 (42%), and during sham reflexology it was 10 out of 22 (46%). Pregnancy rates were 4 out of 26 in the true group and 2 out of 22 in the control group."

Research	Method	Results: Significant Difference	Results: Other Effects
Insomnia (54)	• 13 with sleep disturbance • Control group • Foot reflexology • 6 sessions over 3 weeks	• Produces a clinically important improvement in sleep quality	
Insomnia (87)*+	• 70 insomnia patients • Foot reflexology: twice a day for 10 days • Foot reflexology: once a day for 10 days	• 100% of the twice a day group no longer had a problem sleeping compared to 91% of the once a day group. • Five days after treatment the effective rate was 88% for the twice-a-day group / 22% for the once-a-day group.	
Intestinal function (68)*•	• 32 Healthy men and women • Control group • Foot reflexology • Measured before, during and after	• Increase in the blood flow in the superior mesenteric artery and the subordinate vascular system (the blood flow velocity, the peak systolic and the end diastolic velocities)	
Irritable bowel syndrome (56)	• 28 • Foot reflexology • Mean of 6 sessions	Severe symptoms (abdominal pain, stomach distension and feelings of incomplete evacuation): • 61% lost severe symptoms / a 6% deterioration after 1 month • 39% lost all severe symptoms, others • 21% lost none "Variation in the effectiveness of treatment on clients' severe symptoms was related to their age, temperament and length of time with IBS."	

Research	Method	Results: Significant Difference	Results: Other Effects
Irritable bowel syndrome (55)*•	• 34 • Foot reflexology • Control group (Foot massage) • 30-minute session once a week for 4 weeks, once every two weeks twice • Single blind		No significant difference in: Severity of abdominal pain, constipation or diarrhoea and bloating
Kidney function (69)*•	• 32 Healthy men and women • Control group • Foot reflexology • Measured before, during and after • Double blind	• Systolic peak velocity and end diastolic peak velocity was measured in cm/s, and the resistive index a parameter of the vascular resistance • Decrease of flow resistance in the renal vessels and an increase of renal blood flow. These findings support the hypothesis that organ-associate foot reflexology is effective in changing renal blood flow during therapy	
Kidney stones (74)*	• 30 individuals • Foot reflexology • Control group • Reflexology applied for 5 minutes. For those experiencing pain relief, reflexology continued for 10 more minutes.	• Results: 9 out of the 10 patients in the reflexology group experienced complete pain relief after the treatment which lasted for over an hour and in 5 patients pain was relieved for 4 hours.	

Research	Method	Results: Significant Difference	Results: Other Effects
Kidney and ureter stones (Recovery from lithotrity) (78)+	• 96 individuals following lithtrity • Foot reflexology • Control group • Daily for 30 minutes	• Reflexology group: less pain, began excretion earlier & completed the excretion process earlier • Excretion of fragmented calculus in seven days: Reflexology group, 30; Control group:5. • Fifteen days or less: reflexology group: 43; Control group 22 • Completed excretion in less than 20 days: Reflexology group, all forty-six; Control group, 38	
Knee replacement (Recovery from surgery) (141)*	• 38 post surgical knee replacement patients • Foot reflexology (Morrell Method/ light pressure) applied within 24 hours of surgery and three times a week thereafter • Placebo group (full reflexology session without areas "thought by the reflexologist to influence healing of the knee') • Control group	Patients were assessed for: • Length of stay (strict criteria) • Length of stay (broad criteria) • Total morphine (mg) administered 48-hour post surgically • Average codydrmol (units per day after the 48 hour period)	Results: "There was no significant difference in any of the three groups, with the exception of morphine consumption in the early postoperative period (48 hours after surgery). Patients receiving real or placebo reflexology treatment used significantly less morphine than the control group."

Research	Method	Results: Significant Difference	Results: Other Effects
Lactation in new mothers (96)*+	• 217 new mothers • Foot reflexology (100: 30 hours after giving birth and 17: 30 to 120 hours after) • Control group of 100 • Daily 10 to 15 minutes	• Foot reflexology group: Lactation was initiated in 43.47 hours (+12.39 hours). • Control group: 66.97 hours (+28.16 hours). • At 72 hours satisfactory lactation documented in 98% and 67% of the two groups. • Reflexology work helped avoid use of drugs potentially harmful to the baby	
Leukopenia (Pathologically low white blood cell count) (121)*+	• 47 patients • Foot reflexology (29) • Control group (17)(Pharmacol-therapy) • Daily, 1 month to 2 years (majority between 1 and 2 years)	Symptoms improved: Reflexology group • Upper respiratory tract infection (28 patients):14 symptom free, 26 effectively treated. • Urinary infection (18 patients): 8 symptom free,17 effectively treated •Insomnia(19 patients): 8 symptom free,16 effectively treated • Weakness (24 patients): 8 symptom free, 22 effectively treated Control group: similar for upper respiratory tract, urinary tract infection. Effective for insomnia (71%) / weakness (80%) • White blood cell count improved: 650-3,800 cubic mm. before/ 5,000-7,000 *Continued next page*	

Research	Method	Results: Significant Difference	Results: Other Effects
Continued from previous page		after (12/6 in control-group); 4,000-4,500 cubic mm before / 5,000-8,000 after (12 in reflexology group / 6 in control group); under 4,000 cubic mm. before / 4,000 cubic mm after (5, reflexology group / 6, control group). Treatment ineffective under 4,000 cubic mm (3, reflexology group / 4, control group	
Lower back pain (93)*	• 40 minutes once a week for 6 weeks • Foot reflexology • Sham treatment group • Randomized and blinded	VAS scores for pain reduced in the treatment group by a median value of 2.5 cm, with minimal change in the sham group (0.2 cm).	
Lower back pain (Chronic) (105)*	• 243 participants randomised to one of three groups: • Reflexology • Relaxation • Non-intervention (usual care by GP)	"The quantitative data suggest that reflexology is ineffective for managing CLBP, while the qualitative data suggest otherwise. This incongruence between results raises important questions for the design of research studies into the efficacy of CAMs. Should the patients view of efficacy be negated because 'objective' measures showed no effect? or the appropriateness of the scientific parameters questioned because they are in conflict with patients notion of efficacy?"	• (ANOVA) No significant differences between the groups pre and post treatment on the primary outcome measures of pain $(F(4, 310)=1.152, p=.332)$ and functioning $(F(4, 318)=2.039, p=.132)$ • "Interview data revealed that the majority of participants reported treatment led to reduction in pain, increased relaxation and an enhanced ability to cope."

Research	Method	Results: Significant Difference	Results: Other Effects
Memory (Poor) See Hyperlipimia (85)+			
Menopausal women (37)*•	• 76 • Foot reflexology • Foot massage control group • Same practitioners provided both foot reflexology and foot massage • 45 minutes, 9 times over 19 weeks (once a week for six weeks followed by once a month for three months)	"… reduced menopausal symptoms of anxiety, depression, hot flushes and night sweats by some 30%-50% of what they were at the outset.	"No significant difference between treatment and control group (foot massage)."
Menopausal women (89)+	• 82 women • Foot reflexology (42 women) • Foot reflexology with auricular point magnet adhesion control group (40 women) • Daily for 30 minutes over 60 days	Reflexology group/ Reflexology +auricluar: • 17 (40.48%) / 9 (22.5%): fully recovered;: fully recovered (symptoms disappeared, no relapse at 2 months) • 20 (47.62%) / 16 (40%): significantly recovered (symptoms disappeared, relapse at 2 months but disappeared with more treatment) • 4 (9.25%) / 9 (22.50): effective results (symptoms relieved) • 1 / 6 (15%): ineffective results	

Research	Method	Results: Significant Difference	Results: Other Effects
Menopausal women (12)*^	• 40 • Foot reflexology • Control group • Twice per week for 6 weeks	Statistically significant differences: • Climacteric symptoms (Menopause) • Fatigue • Total cholesterol • Cortisol	No significant difference in: • High density lipoprotein (HDL) • Low density lipoprotein (LDL) • Triglyceride
Mental health (Emotional needs) (88)	• 49 individuals in need of emotional help • once a week for 8 weeks for 30 minutes	Improvement in: • physical aspects • significant improvement in emotional state • improvement in ability to concentrate • increase in motivation for a significant number of participants • significant increase in confidence and self-esteem levels • improvement in communication and ability to articulate ideas more effectively • "importance of being touched during treatment in a safe non-intrusive / abusive manner," • reduction of medication by several	

Research	Method	Results: Significant Difference	Results: Other Effects
Mental health (Severe and enduring) (150)	• 6 individuals (5 with schizophrenia and 1 with bi-polar affective disorder. • 6 foot reflexology sessions over 6 to 12 weeks	• "Qualitative data revealed that reflexology was accepted by the clients in terms of their interest, attendance and tolerance of touch." • "Many of the conversations during and after the reflexology sessions appeared far more meaningful and detailed" • "The conversation for the client seemed more productive in comparison to many key worker/client sessions"	
Mental retardation (95)*+	• 80 children • Foot reflexology • Control group • One to two times a week for a year	Significantly improvement in: • height, weight, health states • social living abilities (increase of 28.20 compared to 21.47 in control group) • intellectual development (IQ change increase of 1.85 years to 57.65 from 55.80)	

Research	Method	Results: Significant Difference	Results: Other Effects
Middle-aged women (3)*•^	• 46 • Self foot reflexology • Outcome variables were measured 4 times, at baseline, pre training, after training, and after the intervention • 2 weeks training followed by daily self foot reflexology for 6 weeks (2 days at the research center, 5 days at home)	Statistically significant difference in: • Depression • Perceived stress • Systolic blood pressure • Natural-killer cells and Ig G (antibodies)	No statistically significant difference in: • Diastolic blood pressure • Pulse • Cortisol
Migraine headache (94)*	• 32 patients • Two times a week for two or three months plus a placebo drug • Fluarizin treatment and massage of a non-specific area twice a week for 12 sessions • Blinded	Reflexology treatment was at least as effective as the Fluarizin treatment and may be classified as an alternative non-pharmacological therapeutic treatment that would be particularly appropriate to those patients that were unable to follow pharmacological treatment.	

Research	Method	Results: Significant Difference	Results: Other Effects
Migraine headache (130)	• 16 female migraine sufferers • Once a week foot reflexology session for 12 women; once a month for two; twice a month for two	• Before sessions women rated their headaches at 8.1 on a scale of 10. After they rated them at 4.43. • 14 of the 16 women reduced or eliminated medication. • Once a week sessions; Before 10 clients experienced a total of 49 to 67 migraines a month. After, 6 women experienced 1 migraine a month, 2 none, 1 two a year and 1 three times a year. Headache averaged a duration of 12.5 to 23.7 hours before and 2.5 to 3 hours after. One woman went from 30 migraines a month with a duration of 2-6 hours to 7 and 2 hours after. One woman went from 30 to 60 migraines a month with a duration of 2-3 days to 30 migraines a month of one-half hour after. • Once a month sessions: 1 women went from two a month to one a month of the same duration; 1 went from once a week to once a month and duration of 1-3 days to 1-2 days. • Twice a month the two women saw no change.	

Research	Method	Results: Significant Difference	Results: Other Effects
Multiple sclerosis (97)*	• 27 multiple sclerosis patients • Foot reflexology • Control group • Once a week for 18 weeks	• 6 weeks: a significant number of people in the treatment group showed an improvement in their symptoms, and most of these improvements were maintained. • 12 weeks: many of the participants had lost some of the improvements • 18 weeks: participants in treatment group saw some improvements in 45% of the symptoms compared to 13% in the control group. • Reflexology does offer some benefit to MS patients especially in the first 6 weeks of treatment; treatment sessions need to be regular; benefits seem to diminish after twelve weeks.	
Multiple sclerosis (167)	• 50 multiple sclerosis patients • Foot reflexology applied by nurse therapists • Cross over design: comparison to progressive muscle relaxation training • 6 weeks with 4 week break followed by 6 weeks of other therapy	• State anxiety (systolic blood pressure, heart rate) values better for reflexology • Cortisol values better for reflexology • Significant difference in both therapies for systolic blood pressure but favoring progressive muscle relaxation	"Limited evidence of difference between two treatments complicated by ordering effects." Problem: Measures were taken pre-treatment series and post-treatment series however: "despite the 4 week break most outcome measures did not return to pre-treatment levels." (ordering)

Research	Method	Results: Significant Difference	Results: Other Effects
Multiple sclerosis (98)*	• 71 patients (53 completed) • Foot reflexology ("manual pressure on specific points in the feet and massage of the calf area") • Sham Control group ("nonspecific massage of the calf area") • 45 minutes once a week for 11 weeks	• Specific reflexology treatment was of benefit in alleviating motor; sensory and urinary symptoms in MS patients • Significant improvement in the differences in mean scores of paresthesias (burning, prickling, itching and tingle) (intensity remained significant at three months of follow-up), urinary symptoms and spasticity for the reflexology group. • Improvement (borderline significance) in mean scores of muscle strength between the reflexology group and the controls ($P = 0.06$).	
Myopia (123)+	• 29 primary school students, lowest level of vision was 0.1 and highest was 1.2 with average of 0.781 • Foot reflexology • Daily, 30-40 minutes for 70 days	Results; • 24 eyes fully recover • 21 eyes significantly effective. • Average eyesight was 1.081, an improvement of 0.3 from before treatment • Children with astymatism (8)*^ improved an average of 0.113 versus 0.371 for those without • Eyesight improved in 3-4 sessions for those with eyesight higher than 1.0	

Research	Method	Results: Significant Difference	Results: Other Effects
Myopia (Adolescent) (119)+	• 34 Middle school students with average visual acuity of 0,27 (right eye) and 0.44 (left eye) • Foot reflexology • 5-10 minutes • 10 times as a course (over 15-30 days)	Total effective rate of 83.8%: After two courses of treatment among the 68 eyes: • 10 (14.7%) showed more than 0. 5 increase in visual acuity • 23 (33.8%) increased by 0.25-0.40 • 24 (35.3%) by 0.1-0.25	
Nervous exhaustion (100)	• 20 patients (chief symptoms were dizziness, insomnia, memory loss, indigestion and headaches) • Foot reflexology • Daily for 7 days	• 40% experienced complete' cure' • 35% had greatly improved • 15% had mildly improved • 10% showed no change at all	
Neurodermatitis (99)*+	• 30 patients • Foot reflexology • Control group • Daily for 10 to 30 days	• Effective rate for the treated group was 46.7% very effective and 53.3% effective. • Control group, 33.3% were very effective, 40% were effective and 26.7 were ineffective. • Reflexology is a simple, effective, economical and lacking the side effects of drugs given the control group (fatigue, sleeplessness, gastrointestinal symptoms, with hormonal dermatitis resulting from long-term use)	

Research	Method	Results: Significant Difference	Results: Other Effects
Neuropathy (Diabetes mellitus (type 2)) (6)*^	• 76 (ages 40-79) • Self foot reflexology • Control • 6 weeks	Good effect: • Improving peripheral neuropathy (especially tingling and pain) • Improving ability to sense 10-g monofilament	Not effective: • Improving peripheral circulation
Osteoarthritis (13)*^	• 41 middle aged women • Foot reflexology • Control group • 30 minutes, 3/week for 4 weeks	Significant improvement in relieving: • Pain • Depression	
Osteoarthritis (144)*	• 119 patients • Foot reflexology • Placebo foot massage • Control (Arthritis information) • 15 minute intervention	• Significantly less posttest pain for groups receiving either reflexology or foot massage • Clinical effect was found in the reflexology group who had 8 to 18% improvement (less pain on all pain scales), compared with those in the massage group.	• Reflexology did not statistically result in less pain than massage. A limitation was the researcher administering all interventions and questionnaires.
Ovulation (164)*	• 48 women • Foot reflexology group (26 women) • Sham reflexology with gentle massage (22 women) • Single-blinded • 8 sessions over 10 weeks		"The rate of ovulation during true reflexology was 11 out of 26 (42%), and during sham reflexology it was 10 out of 22 (46%). Pregnancy rates were 4 out of 26 in the true group and 2 out of 22 in the control group."

Research	Method	Results: Significant Difference	Results: Other Effects
Oxygen saturation, Pulse rate, Respiratory rate (Strength of stimulus) (124)+	• Unknown • Hand reflexology and foot reflexology • 3 times, applied one hour after meals; testing conducted 1/2 hour after reflexology work	• Remarkable and significant results produced by stimulation applied of moderate strength as opposed to low strength • Oxygen saturation rate for moderate strength 20.50 and for low strength 17.17 • Respiratory rate for moderate strength: 98.73 and for low strength: 97.50	
Pain (Threshold and tolerance) (75)	• 16 healthy individuals • Foot reflexology • Cross over design (Subjects participate in Treatment group and then Control group) • Single reflexology session (treatment group) or sham TENS session (Control group) • Immersion of hand in ice to create pain	Following reflexology work and when compared to sham TENS • Significant increase in pain threshold, the time it takes for the subject to find the experience painful • Significant increase in pain tolerance, the time it takes until the subject can no longer keep his/her hand in the ice water "These findings indicate the possibility of using reflexology in the management of pain."	
Pain (Efficacy of Reflexology as a Palliative Treatment in Nursing Home Residents with Dementia) (31)*•	• 80 patients • Foot reflexology • Control group • Pre-test/post-test • 1 / week for 4 weeks, 30 minutes each / 120 minutes	• Significantly greater decrease in physiological measures of stress: blood pressure, heart rate, and salivary measures of cortisol, alpha amyase and DHEA • Significantly greater decrease in pain and depression	

Research	Method	Results: Significant Difference	Results: Other Effects
Pain (Miscellaneous) (76)+	• 60 individuals who were experiencing pain (ages 1 to 73) • Foot reflexology (20 minutes - 40 minutes)	• Following one session 18 of the 60 were healed. 11 were healed following 2 or 3 sessions, 22 were effectively treated after 2 or 3 sessions. Reflexology was ineffective for 9 cases after 1 to 3 sessions	Pain resulted from: Toothache (6), headache (8), sore throat (50), stiff neck (40), shoulder pain/old wound (2), breast pain (2), chest & rib pain (2), dysmenorrhea (3), abdominal pain (5), wrist and leg pain (19), and joint pain in limb
Pain (AIDS) (42)*	• 28 hospitalized AIDS patients • Foot reflexology] • Cross over design • 30 min., 2 reflexology and 2 sham sessions over 4 days	• Significantly less pain and fatigue	"but no significant difference on a 1-item numeric pain intensity scale"
Pain (Birthing/Relieving labor pains) (47)*	• 213 women • Control group (105 women) • Reflexology provided during labor	Reflexology group experienced: • average birth process of 2.48 + 1.48 hours • effective rate (analgesia) was 94.4%	Control group experienced: • average birth process of 3.32 + 1.19 hours
Pain (Birthing/Relieving labor pains) (48)	• 68 women • Reflexology provided during delivery	• 90% effective rate as a pain killer during delivery • 11 of 14 with retention of placenta avoided operation	

Research	Method	Results: Significant Difference	Results: Other Effects
Pain (Blood pressure, pain, control over falls in senior citizens) (25)*•	• 48 senior citizens • Foot reflexology mat walking • Pretest/posttest • Control group • 3 / week for 45 minutes over 8 weeks / 1080 minutes	• Reductions in diastolic blood pressure • Greatly improved perceptions of control over falls • Significantly reduced daytime sleepiness and pain • Increased psychosocial well-being • Considerable improvements ability to perform 'activities of daily living' • Statistically significant change in systolic blood pressure pre-to-post change in systolic blood pressure for the experimental group only, indicating reduced systolic blood pressure	
Pain (Cancer/Pain and anxiety) (21)*•	• 86 patients • Partner delivered foot reflexology • Control group (read a book of their choice to their partner) • Both groups: 30 minutes three times a week, minimum of four weeks	Significant decrease in pain intensity and anxiety	
Pain (Cancer/Pain and nausea) (22)•	• 87 patients • Foot reflexology • 10 minutes	"…significant and immediate effect on the patients' perceptions of pain, nausea and relaxation"	

Research	Method	Results: Significant Difference	Results: Other Effects
Pain (Cancer/ Pain) (57)•	• 36 Inpatients of metastic cancer • Foot reflexology two times 24 hours apart • Pre-test/Post intervention / 3 hours after / 24 hours after	• Positive immediate effect in pain reduction	• No statistically significant effect 3 hours after • No statistically significant effect 24 hours after
Pain (Cance:r Pain management / Pain / Anxiety) (134)•	• 23 breast or lung cancer on an inpatient oncology unit • Foot reflexology • Crossover design • 30 minutes of reflexology one day / 30 minutes of rest on another	• For breast cancer patients, a significant decrease in pain, as measured by the descriptive words of the Short Form-McGill Pain Questionnaire (SF-MPQ); (M=?0.41, SD = 0.71, p =.048) • Significant decrease in anxiety, as measured by the VAS for anxiety, for both breast-cancer patients (n = 13, M =?17.38, \SD = 21.29, p = 0.01) and lung-cancer patients (n = 10,M=?21.6, SD = 25.49, p =.02)	• The Visual Analogue Scale (VAS) for pain and the present pain intensity showed no significant differences between the intervention and control conditions
Pain (Chest pain)(73)	• 4 individuals with chest pain but no cardiac artery disease • 1 per week for 8 weeks	• "Three of the four experienced a complete relief from their original symptoms after nine months and the remaining patient reported a reduction in pain."	

Research	Method	Results: Significant Difference	Results: Other Effects
Pain (Diabetes mellitus (type 2) (6)*^ Peripheral blood circulation, Peripheral neuropathy)	• 76 (ages 40-79) • Self foot reflexology • Control • 6 weeks • Self-help	Good effect: • Improving peripheral neuropathy (especially tingling and pain) • Improving ability to sense 10-g monofilament	Not effective: • Improving peripheral circulation
Pain (Herniated disc/lumbro-sacral) (72)•	• 40 individuals • Foot reflexology • 3 sessions in 1 week	• 62.5% reported a reduction in pain	
Pain (Kidney stones) (74)*	• 30 individuals • Foot reflexology • Control group • Reflexology applied for 5 minutes. For those experiencing pain relief reflexology work continued for another 10 minutes.	• The results showed that 9 out of the 10 patients in the reflexology group experienced complete pain relief after the treatment which lasted for over an hour and in 5 of the patients pain was relieved for 4 hours.	
Pain (Lower back, chronic) (105)*	• 243 participants randomised to one of three groups: • Reflexology • Relaxation or • Non-intervention (usual care by GP)	"The quantitative data suggest that reflexology is ineffective for managing CLBP, while the qualitative data suggest otherwise. This incongruence between results raises important questions for the design of research studies into the efficacy of CAMs. Should the patients view of efficacy be negated because 'objective' measures showed no effect? or the appropriateness of the scientific parameters questioned because they are in conflict with patients notion of efficacy?"	• (ANOVA) No significant differences between the groups pre and post treatment on the primary outcome measures of pain ($F(4, 310)=1.152, p=.332$) and functioning ($F(4, 318)=2.039, p=.132$) • "Interview data revealed that the majority of participants reported treatment led to reduction in pain, increased relaxation and an enhanced ability to cope."

Research	Method	Results: Significant Difference	Results: Other Effects
Pain (Lower back) (93)*	• 40 minutes once a week for 6 weeks	VAS scores for pain reduced in the treatment group by a median value of 2.5 cm, with minimal change in the sham group (0.2 cm).	
Pain (Osteoarthritis) (13)*^	• 41 middle aged women • Foot reflexology • Control group • 30 minutes, 3/ week for 4 weeks 12 sessions/360 minutes	Significant improvement in relieving: • Pain • Depression	
Pain (Phantom limb) (67) •	• 7 men and 3 women with unilateral lower limb amputations and a history of phantom limb pain • 30-week period with weekly pain diaries and: Phase 1: diary for base line of pain. Phase 2: 6 weekly reflexology treatments. Phase: 3 Diary only/ resting phase. Phase 4: 6 weekly teaching sessions. Phase 5: self treatment	Each reflexology treatment, teaching and self-treatment had made a highly significant difference / effective in eradicating or reducing the intensity and duration of phantom limb pain.	

Research	Method	Results: Significant Difference	Results: Other Effects
Pain (Post operative / General surgery) (101)*	• 60 general surgery patients • Foot reflexology • Control group • foot reflexology applied together with standard pain drugs, nonsteroidal anti-inflammatory drugs and opioids (opium-containing drugs) 20 minutes before the measurement time periods (0, 2, 6, and 24 hours)	This study show a decrease of the quantity of pain killers in the foot reflexology group to less than 50% in comparison with control group	
Pain (Post-operative pain and anxiety among cancer patients)(157)*	• 61 patients • Foot reflexology applied on days 2, 3, 4 after surgery for 20 minutes in addition usual pain management • Control group: usual pain management	•" less pain ($P <.05$) and anxiety ($P <.05$) over time were reported by the intervention group compared with the control group" • "intervention group received significantly less opioid analgesics than the control group ($P <.05$)"	
Pain (Post surgical recovery) (82)*	• 130 post gynecological surgery patients • Foot reflexology • Control group • A few days		• Not recommended: occasionally trigger abdominal pain • Various effects, some negative • Foot massage control group more relaxing and positive
Pain (Surgical ward) (172)	• 45 patients • 5 minute hand reflexology applied to each hand	Significant pain relief, improvement in feeling and an increase in skin temperature	

Research	Method	Results: Significant Difference	Results: Other Effects
Pain (Post surgical recovery) (81)*	• 130 post abdominal surgery patients • Foot reflexology • Control group (foot massage) • 15 minutes for 5 days	• More able to void without problems • Indwelling catheter removed earlier	Control (foot massage group): • significant results in the subjective measures of well-being, pain and sleep (slept better)
Pain (Post surgical) (106)*	• 45 post open-heart surgery patients • Group 1: Reflexology with aromatherapy 1st, 2nd, and 3rd day after opened-heart surgery as well as pre-surgery information "Pain relieving after cardiac surgery" • Group 2: pre-surgery information • Group 3: Standard nursing care	• Mean of unpleasant symptoms score in the group receiving preoperative information combined with foot reflexology with aromatherapy was the lowest. • Mean of unpleasant symptoms score in the group receiving preoperative information combined with foot reflexology with aromatherapy was the lowest.	
Pain (Post surgical) (Knee replacement) (141)*	• 38 post surgical knee replacement patients • Foot reflexology (Morrell Method/ light pressure) applied within 24 hours of surgery and three times a week thereafter • Placebo group (full reflexology session without areas "thought by the reflexologist to influence healing of the knee') • Control group	Patients were assessed for: • length of stay (strict criteria) • length of stay (broad criteria) • total morphine (mg) administered 48-hours post surgically • average codydrmol (units per day after the 48 hour period).	Results: "There was no significant difference in any of the three groups, with the exception of morphine consumption in the early postoperative period. Patients receiving real or placebo reflexology treatment used significantly less morphine than the control group."

Research	Method	Results: Significant Difference	Results: Other Effects
Pain (Premenstrual syndrome/ Dysmenorrhea) (15)*^	• 40 female college students • Foot reflexology • Control group • 60 minutes, 6/60 days/ 360 minutes	Relieved symptoms: • Fatigue (50%) • Insomnia (40%) • Abdominal pain (35%) • Lower abdominal pain (30%) • Constipation (30%)	
Pain (Sinusitis) (77)*	• 150 individuals • Three groups performing daily for 2 weeks: Reflexology Irrigation with a bulb syringe Nasal irrigation with a nasal irrigation pot.	• 36 percent of subjects reported decreased use of sinus medication (decongestants, antihistamines, pain relievers, and nasal sprays) • No difference between 3 groups • Reflexology was the control	
Peptic ulcer (156)*+	• 162 individuals • Randomized • Foot reflexology, stomach or duodenum reflex area, two times a day, each for 15 min. to 20 min. for four weeks • Control group: drugs	• Symptoms disappeared 80 cases (97.56%), two "cured" after treatment in 78 patients (95.12%) • Control group, the symptoms disappeared after treatment of 65 cases (81.25%), two "cured" after treatment of 62 cases (77.50%). • Significant between the two groups (P <0.05)	

Research	Method	Results: Significant Difference	Results: Other Effects
Phantom limb pain (67) •	• 7 men and 3 women with unilateral lower limb amputations and a history of phantom limb pain • 30-week period with weekly pain diaries and: Phase 1: diary for base line of pain. Phase 2: 6 weekly reflexology treatments. Phase: 3 Diary only/ resting phase. Phase 4: 6 weekly teaching sessions. Phase 5: self treatment	Each reflexology treatment, teaching and self-treatment made a highly significant difference / effective in eradicating or reducing the intensity and duration of phantom limb pain	
Physiological measure (137)	• 5 volunteers • 10 minute foot reflexology session tested • 20 minute reflexology session tested	• Heart rate, blood pressure: decreased • Carbon dioxide density exhaled from nose: increased 9% • EEG (increase in alpha wave) and ECG (fall in interval ratio) both indicate increase in relaxation • Abdominal respiration rate declined slightly	
Pneumoconiosis (Coal workers') (2)*•^	• 59 coal workers' pneumoconiosis patients • Foot reflexology • Control group • 60 minutes, 2/ week for five weeks 10 sessions/ 600 minutes	Scores decreased significantly in the experimental group but not in the control group for: • Fatigue and insomnia	

Research	Method	Results: Significant Difference	Results: Other Effects
Pneumoconiosis (Coal workers') (1)*^	• 59 coal workers' pneumoconiosis patients • Foot reflexology • Control group • 60 minutes, 2/week for 5 weeks/ 10 sessions/ 600 minutes	Scores decreased significantly in the experimental group but not in the control group for: • Depression and anxiety	
Pneumonia (102)+	• 122 patients • Foot reflexology (reflexology and medication) • Control group (medication) • Daily	• Treatment group 7.8 days average time of treatment with a course of the disease as 10.2 days. The curative rate was 96.5% with improvement in the other 2 cases. • Control group average treatment time of 9.7 days with the total course of the disease at 12.3 days. The curative rate was 92% with 5 cases improved.	
Polycystic ovaries (103)	• 8 women • Foot reflexology • 19 times over 5 to 6 months	• Length of menstrual cycles changed significantly with an average fall of 14.81 days (p = 0,0379). • Number of follicles in the ovaries showed a marginally significant average fall of 16.3 follicles (p = 0,0531).	• Hormone Values and Quality of Life did not show statistical significant changes from before to after the treatment
Post-partum women recovering from Cesarean section (Gastrointestinal function)(163)*	• 194 women • Foot reflexology group (108 cases) • Control group (86 cases) • 3 consecutive days	Significantly difference in time to first defecation for reflexology group	

Research	Method	Results: Significant Difference	Results: Other Effects
Post partum (Urinary system) (160)*+	• 180 inpatients after cesarean section • "Artificial" foot reflexology group • Machine foot reflexology group • Control group	Significantly shorter voiding time for "artificial" foot reflexology group and machine foot reflexology group	
Postpartum Women (159)*+	• 240 Puerperal women 6 hours of work (?): • Group A: foot reflexology with traditional Chinese medicine foot bath • Group B: Chinese medicine foot Bath • Group C: heated foot bath and reflexology no work: • Group D: Control	Results: Group A had a significant difference in: "Appetite, lactation, exhaust, Elu volume, high end of the Palais, intervention; Anxiety, depression score" ($P < 0.01$).	
Postpartum Women (Anxiety and depression) (161)*+	• 240 Puerperal women 6 hours of work (?): • Group A: foot reflexology with traditional Chinese medicine foot bath • Group B: Chinese medicine Foot bath • Group C heated foot bath and reflexology • Group D: Control	Results: Significant difference for foot reflexology with traditional Chinese medicine foot bath group for anxiety and depression score $P < 0.01$	
Postpartum Women (14)*^	• 31 • Foot reflexology • Control group 5 / week for 2 weeks /10 sessions	• Decrease in TG (triglycerides) levels in blood serum	

Research	Method	Results: Significant Difference	Results: Other Effects
Post Patrum (Sleep) (170)*	• 65 women • Foot reflexology • Control group (no intervention) • 30-minute foot reflexology session at the same time each evening for five consecutive days administered by a certified nurse reflexologist	•"an intervention involving foot reflexology in the postnatal period significantly improved the quality of sleep." • "midwives should evaluate maternal sleep quality and design early intervention programmes to improve quality of sleep in order to increase maternal biopsychosocial well-being."	
Post operative (Pain) (101)*	• 60 general surgery patients • Foot reflexology • Control group • 15-20 minutes	Decrease of the quantity of pain killers in the foot reflexology group to less than 50% in comparison with control group	
Post-operative (Pain and anxiety among cancer patients)(157)*	• 61 patients • Foot reflexology applied on days 2, 3, 4 after surgery for 20 minutes in addition usual pain management • Control group: usual pain management	•" less pain ($P < .05$) and anxiety ($P < .05$) over time were reported by the intervention group compared with the control group" • "intervention group received significantly less opioid analgesics than the control group ($P < .05$)"	

Research	Method	Results: Significant Difference	Results: Other Effects
Post surgical pain (143)*	• 40 elderly patients with prostatectomy • Foot reflexology • Control group • Symptom management for pain and frequency of pain medication • One session	• Posttest mean score on pain of an experimental group was significantly lower than of the pretest (X = 7.230, X = 3.75, t=16.335, $p<.001$) • Posttest mean score of pain of an experimental group was significantly lower than of a control group (X = 3.75, X =6.65, t =-10.627, $p<.001$) • Posttest mean score of frequency pain medication taking of an experimental group was significantly lower than of a control group (X = 1.05, X = 1.85, t-=-2.36, $p<.05$)	
Post surgical recovery (107)*	• Foot reflexology • Control group	Reflexology enhances urination, stimulates bowel movements and so aids recovery. • Patients who received reflexology also showed a much less need for medication than patients in the control group	
Post surgical recovery (81)*	• 130 post abdominal surgery patients • Foot reflexology • Control group (foot massage) • 15 minutes for 5 days	• More able to void without problems • Indwelling catheter removed earlier • Slept worse	Foot massage group: significant results in the subjective measures of well-being, pain and sleep.

Research	Method	Results: Significant Difference	Results: Other Effects
Post surgical recovery (82)*	• 130 post gynecological surgery patients • Foot reflexology • Control group (foot massage) • A few days		• Not recommended: Various effects, some negative; occasionally trigger abdominal pain • Foot massage control group more relaxing and positive
Post-traumatic stress disorder (133)	• Unknown number of sessions applied to 75 study participants, victims of community violence in Northern Ireland	• Significant improvements in psychological health and levels of depression over time	• Changes in post-traumatic stress disorder symptom severity were not significant

Research	Method	Results: Significant Difference	Results: Other Effects
Post-traumatic stress disorder (132)	• 15 Israeli soldiers suffering from post traumatic stress disorder (Yom Kippur War, 1973) • 50-60 minutes weekly for 14 weeks (Cycle 1) • (Included 14 of the original 15 patients) 50-60 minutes weekly for 14 weeks (Cycle 2)	Results: Researchers recommend 2 or 3 sessions per week Cycle 1: • Improvements on a scale of 0 (no change)- 4 (very positive change); (Day 1 after treatment / Day 2 after treatment): Depression (3.2/2.2), Outbursts (3.2/2), Muscle tension (2.9/2.2), Concentration level (2.8/2.2), Sleep scores (2.8/2.2) • Improvements on a scale of 0 -5: General feelings (3.7/2.9) • Reduction in medication by 50% (7 individuals/3 of the 7/ 1 of the 3) Day 3: Back as before Cycle 2: (Immediately after treatment / 3 days after treatment) Depression (2.16/1.16), Outbursts (2.79/2.05), Muscle tension (2.83/1.6), Concentration level (1.98/1.05), Sleep scores (2.56/0.64) • Improvements on a scale of 0 -5: General feelings (3.04/1.2) • Reduction in medication by 50% (11 individuals /3 of the 11)	(132a) • Temporary relief from symptoms including anger, depression and muscle tension • Improved sleep patterns, levels of concentration and a lift in overall mood

Research	Method	Results: Significant Difference	Results: Other Effects
Premature infants (162)*+	• 69 premature infants • Foot reflexology • Control group (breast feeding, premature infant care practices)	Significant differences in sleep duration and total sleep time as well as better 7-day and 30-day weight gain	
Premenstrual syndrome (38)*•	• 35 • Foot, hand, ear reflexology • Control group (Placebo reflexology) • 30 minutes, 1/week for 8 weeks	• Significantly greater decrease in 4 measures of premenstrual symptoms	
Premenstrual syndrome/ Dysmenorrhea (15)*^	• 40 female college students • Foot reflexology • Control group • 60 minutes, 6/60 days	Relieved symptoms: • Fatigue (50%) • Insomnia (40%) • Abdominal pain (35%) • Lower abdominal pain (30%) • Constipation (30%)	
Prostate (108)	• 46 men • Foot reflexology • 13 sessions	• 30 participants (65%) reported a reduction in their need to urinate • 31 (67%) reported a better bladder pressure • 37 (80%) reported reduced sexual problems • 28 (60%) reported improvement of their general condition	

Research	Method	Results: Significant Difference	Results: Other Effects
Prostate (Hyperplasia)(110)*+	• 90 Hyperplasia patients • Foot reflexology (30 cases) • Drug therapy (30 cases) • Foot reflexology and drug therapy (30 cases) • 10 sessions	Ultrasound measurement before and after the course of treatment. Criteria for effectiveness: significant effect - the differences >1.5cm., effective -difference=1-1.4cm. Foot reflexology and drug therapy was the most effective and is recommended as a treatment procedure.	
Prostate (Hypertrophy) (109)+	• 50 men (experiencing frequent and urgent nocturnal urination) • Foot reflexology • Thirty minute sessions were applied once or twice a day for 10 to 21 days.	Among the 50 cases: • 10 were "cured," all symptoms disappeared • 5 showed markedly effective, main symptoms disappeared • 30 were effective, symptoms alleviated • 5 were ineffective, no improvement.	
Sinusitis (77)*	• 150 individuals • Three groups performing daily for 2 weeks: Reflexology Irrigation with a bulb syringe Nasal irrigation with a nasal irrigation pot.	• 36% of subjects in reflexology and irrigation groups reported decreased use of sinus medication (decongestants, antihistamines, pain relievers, and nasal sprays) • No difference between 3 groups • Reflexology was the control	
Sleep (Sleep disturbance, depression disorder, and the physiological index (39)*•+	• 50 elderly women • Foot reflexology • Control group • Pre-test/Post-test • 12 sessions, 30 minutes per session	• Improved sleep quality • Less depression disorder • Higher serotonin levels	

Research	Method	Results: Significant Difference	Results: Other Effects
Sleep (Elderly women) (16)*^	• 100 elderly women • Foot reflexology • Control group • 45 minutes for 3 consecutive days/ 135 minutes	• Sleep score higher • Fatigue score lower • Both scores changed as foot reflexology sessions increased	
Sleep (Pneumoconiosis (Coal workers')) (2)*•^	• 59 coal workers' pneumoconiosis patients • Foot reflexology • Control group • 60 minutes, 2/ week for five weeks 10 sessions/ 600 minutes	Scores decreased significantly in the experimental group but not in the control group for: • Fatigue and insomnia	
Sleep and fatigue (Nurses) (9)*^	• 40 nurses • Self foot reflexology • Control group • 40 minutes, 2/ week for 4 weeks	• Score of fatigue decreased • Score of sleep states increased	
Sleep (Insomnia) (87)*+	• 70 insomnia patients • Foot reflexology: twice a day for 10 days • Foot reflexology: once a day for 10 days	• 100% of the twice a day group no longer had a problem sleeping compared to 91% of the once a day group. • Five days after treatment, however, the effective rate was 88% for the twice-a-day group and 22% for the once-a-day group.	

Research	Method	Results: Significant Difference	Results: Other Effects
Stress (166)	• 48 mothers staying with hospitalized children • Bamboo stepping with a stretching and exercise program practiced in hospital *Bamboo stepping a favorite part for effects and portability*	• Normalization of blood pressure (decreased for high; increased for low) • "Exhilaration" and "feeling good" 24 (50.0%) • "Alleviation of health conditions" expressed in such words as "relief from sore and pain" or "feeling easier with the body" 11 (22.9%) • new "awareness" of "feeling better by moving one's body rather than not moving" 2 (4.2%)	Complaints before participation in program: "physical pain, 27 (56.3%); stiff shoulders, 27 (56.3%); malaise/ exhaustion 13, (27.1%); insomnia, 8,(16.7%); constipation 3, (6.3%), and sensitivity to cold temperatures 3, (6.3%)
Stroke (18)*^	• 31 hospitalized stroke patients • Foot reflexology • Control group • 40 minutes, 2/week for 6 weeks	• Improvement in ADL (activities of daily living) • Less physical, psychological and neuro-sensory fatigue	
Stroke (125)+	• 38 stroke patients • Once a day in first course; every other day in second course; once or twice a week in third course (Course =10 sessions; work continued for some until results were achieved)	Results • 28 cases (74%, symptoms relieved (able to walk independently) • 8 cases (21%) fundamentally recovered (negative Babinski)	

Research	Method	Results: Significant Difference	Results: Other Effects
Students: Constipation, anxiety, depression (19)*^	• 61 nursing students • Foot reflexology • Control group • 2 weeks education on theory; 4 weeks practical skill education, 3 weeks session	• Anxiety states decreased • Bowel function improved • Depression states decreased	
Thyroid (171)	• 9 patients in remission state of thyroid disease • Foot reflexology • Twice a week for 6 weeks	Significant improvement in subjective symptoms: Headache; concentration; cold intolerance; dryness of skin; discomfort and dryness of ocular region; irritability, edema, dizziness, anxiety; urinary frequency; coldness of hands and feet; fatigue No significant change in levels of thyroid hormones (T3, T4, TSH, Free T4)	
Urinary tract infection (112)*+	• 24 cases • Foot reflexology and drug therapy • Control group: drug therapy only • Daily	Treatment group: • 5 showed immediate amelioration of disappearance of symptoms • 7 showing amelioration or disappearance on the second day Control group: • 4 showed amelioration or disappearance on the second day • 8 showed amelioration or disappearance on the third day.	

Research	Method	Results: Significant Difference	Results: Other Effects
Urinary tract stones (Lithotrity) (78)+	• 96 individuals following lithtrity • Foot reflexology • Control group • Daily for 30 minutes	• Excretion of fragmented calculus in seven days: Reflexology group, 30; Control group: 5. • Fifteen days or less: Reflexology group: 43; Control group 22. • Completed excretion in less than 20 days: Reflexology group, all forty-six; Control group, 38	
Urinary tract stones (111)+	• 34 individuals with urinary tract stones • Foot reflexology • 3-20 sessions	"Cure rate" achieved by application of: • 3-5 times for three individuals • 6-8 times for eight individuals • 10-12 times for eight individuals • more than 20 times for 5 individuals.	
Urination (Prostate (Hypertrophy)) (109)+	• 50 men (experiencing frequent and urgent nocturnal urination • Foot reflexology • Thirty minute sessions were applied once or twice a day for 10 to 21 days.	Among the 50 cases: • 10 were "cured," all symptoms disappeared • 5 showed markedly effective, main symptoms disappeared • 30 were effective, symptoms alleviated • 5 were ineffective, no improvement.	

See also Incontinence

Research	Method	Results: Significant Difference	Results: Other Effects
Uroshesis (113)*+	• 40 cases who could not urinate following brain or cranium surgery • Foot reflexology for 30 minutes • Control group (listening to the sound of flowing water, massage applied to the urinary bladder and other conditional reflexes were applied)	Reflexology group: • 65% of the treatment group could excrete urine within 10 minutes; 25% could excrete urine but not completely within 10 to 30 minutes; 10% were unable to urinate 30 minutes Control group: • 30% could excrete urine within 10 minutes; 45% could excrete urine but not completely within 10 to 30 minutes; 25% of the control group were unable to urinate 30 minutes	

Chapter Four

Physiologic Measures, Dosing and Results

Key
* Controlled study
• PubMed (National Institute of Health)
^ Published in a peer-reviewed journal (Korea)
+ Published in a peer reviewed journal (China)

Physiologic Measures, Dosing and Results

Physiologic Measure	Results and Frequency
Alpha amyase	*Foot Reflexology* **Statistically significant reduction physiologic distress as measured by alpha amylase** • 1 / week for 4 weeks, 30 minutes each (Dementia / Nursing home residents) (31)*• Physiologic stress was assessed using blood pressure, heart rate, and salivary measures of cortisol, alpha amyase (sensitive to psycho-social stress) and DHEA
Blood pressure	*Foot Reflexology* **Significant difference** • Daily for 30-40 days: Blood pressure/heart rate: reflexotherapy group (before): +185/80 / 86-74 and (after): +160/75 / 72-70 Blood pressure/heart rate: pharmacotherapy group (before): +180/80 / 78-72 and (after): +160/80 / 76-70 (Coronary heart disease patients) (30)*+ • Twice a week for 6 weeks (Foot reflexology)/ Twice a week for 4 weeks (Self foot reflexology) (Hypertensive patients) (11)*•^ **Significantly greater decrease** • Once per week for 4 weeks, 30 minutes each (Nursing home residents) (31)*• **Decrease** • 20 minutes; 10 minutes (Healthy volunteers) (137) • Twice a week for 6 weeks (Elderly with hypertension) (8)*^ **Lowered** • 1 session (Senior citizens) (28)• • Real time Before: 146 mmHg. fell to about 130 mmHg. after work (Healthy volunteers) (137) **No significant difference** • After one session when foot reflexology compared to foot massage (Healthy individuals) (26)*
	Hand Reflexology • 10 minutes, five times over 3 days Decreased significantly on the 1st session, but not 5th session. (Hemodialysis patients) (40)*

Physiologic Measure	Results and Frequency
Blood pressure (Systolic)	*Foot Reflexology* **Significant difference** • 60 minutes, (Healthy volunteers) (41)*• • 1 session (Cancer patients/chemotherapy) (5)*^ • Pre-test/Post-test; SBP (p=.009)(Cancer chemotherapy patients) (42)* **Decrease in** • Twice per week for 6 weeks / 12 sessions (Elderly with hypertension) (8)*^ **Lowered significantly** • 30 minutes / 5 days (Coronary artery bypass patients) (29)*• • 30 - 40 days; 185/80 before and 160/75 after reflexology: 180/80 before and 160/80 after pharmacotherapy control group (Coronary heart disease patients) (30)*+ **Significantly lower:** • 10 minutes, 5 days a week for one week (Cancer) (Hand reflexology) (152)*
	Self Foot Reflexology **Statistically significant difference**: • Daily for 6 weeks (Middle-aged women) (3)*•^ • Foot reflexology twice per week for 6 weeks; Self foot reflexology twice per week for 4 weeks (Hypertensive patients) (11)*•^
Blood pressure (Diastoli)c	*Foot Reflexology* **Significant difference** • Pre-test/Post-test; DBP (p=.014) (Cancer / chemotherapy patients) (42)* **Significant decrease** • 1 session (Cancer patients/chemotherapy) (5)*^ • 30-40 days; 185/80 before and 160/75 after reflexology: 180/80 before and 160/80 after pharmacotherapy control group (Coronary heart disease patients) (30)*+ **No significant difference** • 60 minutes (Healthy individuals) (41)*• • Twice a week for six weeks, as well as self administered foot reflexology twice a week for four weeks. (Hypertension in the elderly) (8)*^ **No significant changes** • 30 minutes / 5 days (Coronary artery bypass patients) (29)*• **Not significantly lower** • 10 minute daily for 5 days, one week (Cancer) (Hand reflexology) (152)*

Physiologic Measure	Results and Frequency
	Self Foot Reflexology **Reductions in diastolic blood pressure** • Foot reflexology mat walking, three times per week for 45 minutes over 8 weeks (25)*• **No statistically significant difference** • Daily for 6 weeks (Middle-aged women) (3)*•^ • Foot reflexology 2 / week for 6 weeks; Self foot reflexology 2 / week for 4 weeks (Hypertensive patients) (11)*•^
Blood uric acid level	*Foot Reflexology* **Normalized** • 30 minutes, 7 - 10 sessions (Gout) (115)*+
Carbon dioxide (Exhaled)	*Foot Reflexology* **Increased 9%** Carbon dioxide density exhaled from nose (Healthy volunteers) (137)
Carbon dioxide density	*Foot Reflexology* Gas exhaled from the nose, Before: 5.6%; After 6.1%, Increase of 9%. After work, level returned to first measure (Healthy volunteers) (137)
Cholesterol	*Foot Reflexology* **Remarkable reduction** • 30-40 minutes 5 or 6 times a week (High cholesterol patients) (83)+ **Remarkable reduction in cholesterol** • 30-40 minute session five or six times a week for 20 sessions (Hyperlipimia patients) (84)* **Marked statistical difference and reduction** • 30 to 40 minutes daily for 12 days (except Sunday) (High cholesterol patients) (85)+ **Not significantly decreased** (total cholesterol level, HDL and LDL cholesterol) • Twice a week for six weeks, as well as self administered foot reflexology twice a week for four weeks. High density lipoprotein; Low density lipoprotein (Hypertension in the elderly) (8)*^

Physiologic Measure	Results and Frequency
Cortisol	*Foot Reflexology* **Significantly greater decrease** • Once a week for 4 weeks, 30 minutes each (Dementia / Nursing home residents) (31)*• **Statistically significant differences** • Twice a week for 6 weeks (Menopausal women) (12)*^ **Difference** • Once a week for 6 weeks (Multiple sclerosis patients) (167) **No significant difference** • 60 minutes (Healthy volunteers) (41)*• • Weekly for 8 weeks (Post surgical cancer) (168)*
	Self Foot Reflexology **No significant difference** • Daily for 6 weeks (Middle-aged women) (3)*•^
Doppler sonogram	*Foot Reflexology* **Improvement in:** • 1 session (blood flow rate, time, acceleration in lower limbs) (Diabetes) (35)* **Increase in** • Real time blood flow (Intestines) (68)*• **Effective in changing:** • Real time blood flow during therapy (Kidney) (69)*•
ECG	*Foot Reflexology* **Improved remarkably** • ECG: 30-40 days (Coronary heart disease patients) (30)*+ **Relaxation** • Real time (Healthy volunteers) (137) **Change in T-waves** • Real time/Disappearance of angina symptoms (Angina patient) (62)+
	Self Foot Reflexology **Changed significantly** • Real time 20 minutes (Electric foot massager) (63)

Physiologic Measure	Results and Frequency
EEG	*Foot Reflexology* **Significant increases in one or more patterns** • Real time: Significant increase: alpha amplitude, theta amplitude,% alpha synchrony and% theta synchrony (Healthy volunteers) (64) **Increase in relaxation waves** • Real time: increase in alpha frequencies in the brain waves (Healthy volunteers) (66)• • Real time increase in alpha waves that remained following work (Healthy volunteers) (137)
	Hand Reflexology **Increase in relaxation waves** • Real time: Brings the brain-mind mechanism to a lower dimensional chaos indicating a state of 'order out of disorder' (65)•
fMRI	*Foot Reflexology* • Reflexology stimulus applied to lateral inner big toe (left foot) activated reflected region of the brain, the right temporal lobe (127) • Reflexology stimulus applied to eye reflex area showed visual cerebral cortex not activated but reflex area stimulation matched same results as when acupoint stimulated in stroke patients with vision deficits (128) • Reflexology and acupuncture stimuli resulted in activation in the same area of the brain, the insula demonstrating that both at the point (adrenal gland / K1 used for psychological asthma for both) probably regulate emotional and pain effects. The strongest activation in the brain for pressure applied to the adrenal gland reflex area was the insula with functions of homeostasis, pain, emotions) (129) • Stimualtion to the eye, shoulder and small intestine reflex areas resulted in activation of the somatosenory area corresponding to the foot as well as the eye, shoulder and small intestine (visceral and cutaneal/trunk) (169)
Free radicals	*Foot Reflexology* **No difference from control group (Sham reflexology: not applied to symptom appropriate reflex areas)** • 30-40 min. for 10 days: (SOD: increase; GP: increase; GHtal, MDA: decrease) (Healthy/various illness)(51)*+ **Significant difference** • 30-40 min. for 12 days: (SOD, GHtal, MDA) (Cervical spondylosis)(50)*+
Human growth hormone	*Foot Reflexology* **No statistically significant difference** • Weekly for 8 weeks (Post surgical breast cancer patiens) (168)*

Physiologic Measure	Results and Frequency
Immune system	*Foot Reflexology* **Fewer B lympo-cytes** • Weekly for 8 weeks (Post surgical breast cancer) (168)*
	Hand Reflexology • 10 minutes, five / week for five weeks/ 250 minutes: **Increase in lympho-cyte subsets; CD32, CD33, CD34;** "However, **no significant differences** between (experimental and control) groups were found for:CD4 increased significantly (Hemodialysis patients) (10)*^ NK (Natural killer) cells **decreased significantly** and CD 8 **decreased** • 10 minutes, five times over 3 days: Suppressor T cell and NK (Natural killer) cell showed **significant decrease** after the program, but **no significant differences** between the groups. (Hemodialysis patients) (40)*
	Self Foot Reflexology **Statistically significant** difference in: • Daily for 6 weeks (Natural-killer cells and Ig G antibodies) (Middle-aged women) (3)*•^
Intestinal function	*Foot Reflexology* **Increase in:** • Real time Blood flow rate measured before, during and after work (69)*
Kidney function	*Foot Reflexology* **Effective in changing:** • Real time blood flow rate measured before, during and after work (68)*•
	Hand Reflexology **Significant difference:** • 10 minutes, five times over 3 days: BT decreased significantly on both of the 1st and the 5th application; pulse rate and blood pressure were decreased significantly on the 1st times, but not 5th times; Hb (hemoglobin) levels significantly increased (Hemodialysis and cancer patients) (40)* • 10 minutes, five / week for five weeks: Increase in Hb (hemoglobin); Decrease in BUN (blood urea nitrogen) and Cr. (creatinine) (Hemodialysis patients) (10)*^
Melatonin	*Foot Reflexology* **No significant difference from control group**: • 60 minutes (Healthy volunteers) (41)*•
Oxygen density	*Foot Reflexology* **Real time**: Before: 95-97%; during, increase to 97% (Healthy volunteers) (137)

Physiologic Measure	Results and Frequency
Pancreas function	*Foot Reflexology* **Improvement in:** • Blood flow rate in feet measured before, during and after work (Diabetes) (35)* • Daily for 30 days **Greatly reduced**: fasting blood glucose levels; platelet aggregation; length and wet weight of the thrombus; senility symptom scores; serum lipid peroxide (LPO) (Diabetics) (33)*•+ • Daily for 30 days **Marked improvement**. effective rate for 67% in: senility, thrombocyte aggregation rates (TAR), the length and wet weights of thrombosis in vitro, and the serum oxidative lipids (Diabetics) (34)*+
Pulse rate	*Foot Reflexology* **Significant difference** • 60 minutes (Healthy individuals) (41)*• • 1 / week for 4 weeks, 30 minutes each (Nursing home residents) (31)*• • Pre-test/Post-test; Pulse Rate (p=.015) (Cancer chemotherapy patients) (42)* **Decreased** • 20 minutes; 30 minutes (Physiological measures) (137) **Lowered** • 1 session (Senior citizens) (28)• • 30-40 days Pulse Rate 86-74 before and 76-70 after reflexology; 78-72 before and 76-70 after pharmacotherapy control group (Coronary heart disease patients) (30)*+ • Real time: Before, 62; during work on right foot, 54; after work on left foot, 50 (Healthy volunteers) (137)
	Hand Reflexology **Decreased significantly** on the 1st times, but not 5th times. • 10 minutes, five times over 3 days (Hemodialysis patients) (40)* **Lowered** • 10 minutes daily for 5 days (Cancer) (Hand reflexology) (152)*
	Self Foot Reflexology **No statistically significant difference** • Daily for 6 weeks (Middle-aged women) (3)*•^
Prolactin	*Foot Reflexology* **No significant difference** • Weekly for 8 weeks (Post surgical breast cancer patients) (168)*
Serotonin	*Foot Reflexology* **Higher serotonin levels than control group** • 30 minutes, 12 sessions (Elderly women) (39)*•+

Physiologic Measure	Results and Frequency
Triglycerides	*Foot Reflexology* **Decrease in:** • Foot reflexology twice a week for six weeks; Self foot reflexology twice a week for 4 weeks (Hypertension) (11)*•^ • 5 times a week for 2 weeks (Postpartum women) (14)*^ **Strong effect** • 30-40 minutes 5 or 6 times a week (High cholesterol patients) (83)+ **Significantly decreased** • Twice a week for six weeks, as well as self administered foot reflexology twice a week for four weeks. (Hypertension in the elderly) (8)*^ **No change** • Twice a week for 6 weeks (Menopausal women) (12)*^ • 50 minute twice week for 4 weeks (Hypertension) (58)*
	Self Foot Reflexology **Decrease in:** • Foot reflexology twice a week for 6 weeks; Self foot reflexology twice a week for 4 weeks (Hypertension) (11)*•^
Uric acid	*Foot Reflexology* Blood uric acid normalized, 7-10 sessions (Gout) (115)*+
White blood cell count	*Foot Reflexology* White blood cell count improved: 650-3,800 cubic mm before and 5,000-7,000 after (12 in reflexology group and 6 in pharmacotherapy group); from 4,000-4,500 cubic mm before and 5,000-8,000 after (12 in reflexology group and 6 in pharmacotherapy group); from under 4,000 cubic mm before and 4,000 cubic mm after (5 in the reflexology group and 6 of the pharmacotherapy group). • One month to one - two years (Leukopenia)(121)*+

Chapter Five

Effects on Physiological Processes

Key
* Controlled study
• PubMed (National Institute of Health)
^ Published in a peer-reviewed journal (Korea)
+ Published in a peer reviewed journal (China)

Effects on Physiological Processes

Testing Method	Research Details	Significant Effects	Other Effects
Doppler (Intestines)(68)*•	• 32 Healthy men and women • Control group • Foot reflexology • Measured before, during and after	• Increase in the blood flow in the superior mesenteric artery and the subordinate vascular system (the blood flow velocity, the peak systolic and the end diastolic velocities)	
Doppler (Kidney) (69)*•	• 32 Healthy men and women • Control group • Foot reflexology • Measured before, during and after	• Systolic peak velocity and end diastolic peak velocity was measured in cm/s, and the resistive index a parameter of the vascular resistance • Decrease of flow resistance in the renal vessels and an increase of renal blood flow. These findings support the hypothesis that organ-associate foot reflexology is effective in changing renal blood flow during therapy	
Doppler (Circulation in Diabetes mellitus (Type 2)) (35)*	• 20 diabetic/15 healthy • Foot reflexology • Doppler sonagraphic pre-test/Post-test • 1 session	Improvement in blood flow rate, time and acceleration	

Testing Method	Research Details	Significant Effects	Other Effects
fMRI (127) (Frontal lobe activation)	• 10 healthy subjects • Apply reflexology stimulation to inner lateral corner of the left great toe to see if this would activate the part of the brain reflected by this reflex area, the right temporal lobe	Activation of brain: • Temporal lobe (strongest) (Sensory pathways and/or memory, auditory or language functions) • Cerebellum (Motor-sensory pathway) • Right claustrum (secondary somatosensory cortex) • Right anterior central gyrus (Tactile stimulation and movement of toe during work)	
fMRI (129) (Adrenal gland reflex area stimulation compared to acupuncture K1 (comparable acupoint))	• 14 healthy males • pressure applied to adrenal gland reflex area • electrical stimulation of K1 acupoint • Hypothesis: reflex area stimulation would activate the same brain region as acupuncture stimulation; selected area of left foot (adrenal gland reflex area and K1) is related to emotional disorder and pain (adrenal gland and K1 are utilized to work with psychological asthma)	Activation in the insula demonstrated by reflexology or acupuncture stimuli at the point (adrenal gland / K1) probably regulate emotional and pain effects. Activation of brain by reflexology (adrenal gland reflex area): • Insula (Homeostasis, pain, emotions) (Strongest activation) • Homunculus of the cerebral cortex (Sensory) • Parietal lobe (Premotor) Activation of brain by acupuncture (K1 acupoint) • Homunculus (Sensory) • Insula (Homeostasis, pain, emotions) • Working memory	

Testing Method	Research Details	Significant Effects	Other Effects
fMRI (128) (Vision)	• 10 healthy volunteers • Apply reflexology technique applied to left foot, eye reflex area at bases of second and third toes to see if this would activate the visual cerebral cortex	Activation of brain: • Left frontal lobe (Strongest activation) (Polysensory / Premotor area/Language related movement (writing)) • Cerebellum (Conduct impulses to cerebral cortex / Posture, balance, coordination of movements) • Left insula	Visual cerebral cortex not activated but reflex area stimulation matched results when acupoint stimulated in stroke patients with vision deficits: activation of frontal lobe and insula
fMRI (Eye, shoulder, small intestine reflex areas) (169)	• 25 healthy subjects • Reflexology stimulation applied by stick to eye, shoulder and stomach reflex areas	Resulted in activation in the brain of "somatosensory areas corresponding to the foot but also the somatosensory areas corresponding to the eye, shoulder and small intestine (both visceral and cutaneous trunk) or neighboring body parts"	
ECG (Heart rate variability) (62)	• 20 individuals • Electric foot roller • Real time for 20 minutes • Heart rate variability (HRV) signal was measured by three means: correlation dimension analysis (CD), entropy and Poincare plot geometry (SD2(ms)	• Most of the cases under study have changed significantly due to the effect of reflexological stimulation • Measurement by ECG showed a moderate improvement of cardiac function of the heart's activity	

Testing Method	Research Details	Significant Effects	Other Effects
ECG (71)	• 3 Individuals • Electrical stimulation to simulate reflexology work	"Under reflexology, the complexity (quantified by dimension) of the dynamics was lower compared to without reflexologic stimulations with a general drop as degree of stimulation increased. … "This implies that dynamics become less complex and the horizon of predictability increase during reflexology."	
EEG (64)	• 11 individuals • Foot reflexology session • Real time	• 10 of 11 showed significant increases, over the course of the session, in one or more of the following measures: alpha amplitude, theta amplitude,% alpha synchrony and% theta synchrony • "Additionally, and perhaps more importantly, there was a substantial drop in these measures immediately following the baseline period when the hands on portion of the session began."	

Testing Method	Research Details	Significant Effects	Other Effects
EEG (65)•	• 8 individuals • "Reflexological stimulation of the brain reflex area of the hand" (pressure applied to upper half of thumb) • Real time	"We conclude that reflexological stimulation, from the signals and systems point of view bring the brain-mind mechanism to a lower dimensional chaos indicating a state of 'order out of disorder'... "We expected this, as reflexology claims to de-stress and bring relaxation to the brain."	
EEG (66)•	• 30 subjects • Control group (Classical music followed by rock music) • Foot reflexology • Both compared to resting state	Both groups compared to resting state: the number of parallel functional processes active in the brain is less and the brain goes to a more relaxed state. This gives rise to the increase in alpha frequencies in the brain waves	
EEG (70)	• 2 Subjects • "Electrical stimulation to simulate reflexology work was applied to the brain reflex 'point' on the thumbs"	• "Results showed that there was a clear differences in characteristics of EEG signals with and without reflexology. Results signal relaxation effect of reflexology: Under reflexology stimulation frequency components are below 30Hz. Normal EEG signal (50-60Hz)"	

Testing Method	Research Details	Significant Effects	Other Effects
Pain (Threshold and tolerance) (75)	• 16 healthy individuals • Foot reflexology • Cross over design (Subjects participate in Treatment group and then Control group) • Single reflexology session (treatment group) or sham TENS session (Control group) • Immersion of hand in ice to create pain	Following reflexology work and when compared to sham TENS • Significant increase in pain threshold, the time it takes for the subject to find the experience painful • Significant increase in pain tolerance, the time it takes until the subject can no longer keep his/her hand in the ice water "These findings indicate the possibility of using reflexology in the management of pain."	

Chapter Six

Systems of the Body, Dosing and Results

Key

* Controlled study
• PubMed (National Institute of Health)
^ Published in a peer-reviewed journal (Korea)
+ Published in a peer reviewed journal (China)

Systems of the Body, Dosing and Results

System of the Body	Results
Cardio vascular system	**Pulse rate and blood pressure:** Reduced (Real time) (Healthy volunteers) (41)*•; (Senior citizens) (28)•; (Cancer) (151)•
	Blood pressure: Significant difference, daily for 30-40 days (30)*+; Once per week for 4 weeks (31)*• **Systolic blood pressure:** Significant difference, 60 minutes (41)*•; 1 session (5)*^; 10 minutes/day for 3 days; Decrease in, twice a week for 6 weeks (8)*^; Lowered significantly, 30 minutes a day for 5 days (29)*•; Self foot reflexology daily for 6 weeks (3)*•^ **Diastolic blood pressure:** Significant difference, 1 session (42)*; Significant decrease, 1 session (5)*^; Daily for 30-40 days (30)*+; Decrease in twice a week for 6 weeks; No significant difference (41)*•; No significant changes 30 minutes per day for 5 days (29)*•; Self help reflexology Reductions, 3 times per week for 45 minutes for 8 weeks (25)*•; No statistically significant difference, daily for 6 weeks (3)*•^; twice a week for 4 weeks with foot reflexology twice a week for 6 weeks (11)*•^ **Pulse rate:** Significant difference, 60 minutes (41)*•; once per week for 4 weeks for 30 minutes (31)*•; Lowered, 1 session (28)•; daily for 30-40 days (30)*+; Self help foot, No significant difference daily for 6 weeks (3)*•^
Digestive system	**Blood flow to:** Improved (Real time) (68)*• **Constipation:** Improved 10 days, daily (Elderly) (59)*+; 12 weeks (Children) (61)*; 15 sessions (Women) (60)
	Cholesterol: Remarkable reduction, 5 days a week, 20 sessions (84)*; 30-40 minutes daily for 12 days; No significant decrease: twice per week for 6 weeks (11, 8, 12); twice per week for 5 weeks (58)*
	Gout: Relieved 100% of symptoms, 30 minutes, 7 - 10 sessions (115)*+
	Peptic ulcers: Symptoms disappeared for 97.5%; two times a day, each for 15 min to 20 min for four weeks (156)*+

| Endocrine system | **Birthing;** Labor time reduced, During delivery (47)*, During pregnancy, 10 sessions (46); No difference 4 or more sessions (45)*•
Diabetes: Change in blood sugar levels, daily for 30 days (33)*•+ (34); No result 3 per week (7)*^
Menopause: Symptoms disappeared, daily for 60 days (89)+; Symptoms reduced, twice a week for 6 weeks (12)*^; "Reduced menopausal symptoms of anxiety, depression, hot flushes and night sweats by some 30%-50% of what they were at the outset", once a week for six weeks followed by once a month for three months (37)*•
Polycystic ovaries: Length of menstrual cycles changed significantly with an average fall of 14.81 days (p = 0,0379); Number of follicles in the ovaries showed a marginally significant average fall of 16.3 follicles (p = 0,0531). 19 times over 5 to 6 months (103)
Postpartum women:
• Significantly difference in time to first defecation for reflexology group, three consecutive days (Women recovering from Cesarean section/Gastrointestinal function) (163)*
• Significantly shorter voiding time for "artificial" foot reflexology group and machine foot reflexology group, Unknown (Women recovering from Cesarean section/Urinary system)(159)*+
• Foot reflexology with traditional Chinese medicine foot bath group had a significant difference in: "appetite, lactation, exhaust, Elu volume, high end of the Palais, intervention; anxiety, depression score," 6 hours (158)*
• Significant difference for foot reflexology with traditional Chinese medicine foot bath group for anxiety and depression score, 6 hours (160)*+
• Decrease in TG (triglycerides) levels in blood serum, 5 / week for 2 weeks (14)*^
Premenstrual syndrome: Significantly greater decrease in premenstrual symptoms (38%); Relieved symptoms of fatigue (50%), insomnia (40%), abdominal pain (35%), lower abdominal pain (30%), constipation (30%) (15)*^
Prostate: (65%) reported a reduction in their need to urinate; (67%) reported a better bladder pressure; (80%) reported reduced sexual problems; (60%) reported improvement of their general condition (108) |
|---|---|

Immune system	• **CD32, CD33, CD34;Increase in lymphocyte subsets;** "However, **no significant differences** between groups were found for: CD4 increased significantly NK (Natural killer) cells **decreased significantly** and CD 8 **decreased** 10 minutes, five / week for five weeks/ 250 minutes (Hemodialysis patients) (10)*^ • Suppressor T cell and NK (Natural killer) cell showed **significant decrease** after the program, but **no significant differences** between the groups, 10 minutes, five times over 3 days (Hemodialysis patients) (40)* • NK (Natural killer) cells and Ig G antibodies **Statistically significant** difference Daily for 6 weeks (3)*•^ • **White blood cell count**: More effective than medication; 87% improved to normal range, Daily for one month to 1-2 years (121)*+ • **B lympho-cytes** Fewer. Weekly for 8 weeks (Post surgical breast cancer) (168)*
Nervous System	• **Relaxation**: creation of brain waves indicating relaxation as measured by EEG (64) (65)• (66)• • **Activation in the brain** of area reflected by big toe (temporal lobe) and cerebellum (127) • **Activation in the brain** of vision-related areas, cerebellum and primary motor area (128) • **Activation in the brain** of emotional, homeostatic, pain center and sensory motor cortex (129) • **Multiple sclerosis**: Significant number of people in the treatment group showed an improvement in their symptoms and most of these improvements were maintained. (97)* • **Multiple sclerosis**: Specific reflexology treatment was of benefit in alleviating motor; sensory and urinary symptoms in MS patients. (98)* • **Stroke**: Improvement in activities of daily living; Less physical, psychological and neurosensory fatigue (18)*^ • **Stroke**: 28 cases (74%, symptoms relieved (able to walk independently); 8 cases (21%) fundamentally recovered (negative Babinski) (Stroke) (125)+
Respiratory system	**Asthma**: Disappearance of symptoms, daily for 2 to 12 weeks (142)*+; No difference from control group, 60 minutes per week for 10 weeks (139)*•; Reflexology and control groups both showed decrease in consumption of beta-2-agonists and increase in peak-flow levels (44)*• **Oxygen saturation rate**: Increased (124)+ **Pneumonia**: Treatment group 7.8 days average time of treatment with a course of the disease as 10.2 days. Curative rate was 96.5% with improvement in the other 2 cases. (102)+ **Respiratory rate**: Impacted (124)+

Skeletal system	**Knee replacement** (Recovery from surgery): Less morphine for 48 hours post-operatively; No difference in hospital stay or pain-killer after 48 hours (141)* **Lower back pain**: Scores for pain reduced in the treatment group by a median value of 2.5 cm, with minimal change in the sham group (0.2 cm). (93)* **Lower back pain (chronic)**: No significant differences between the groups pre and post treatment on the primary outcome measures of pain; "Interview data revealed that the majority of participants reported treatment led to reduction in pain, increased relaxation and an enhanced ability to cope." (105)* **Osteoarthritis**: Significant improvement in relieving pain and depression (13)*^ **Osteoarthritis**: Significantly less posttest pain for groups receiving either reflexology or foot massage) (144)* **Phantom limb pain**: Each reflexology treatment, teaching and self-treatment had made a highly significant difference / effective in eradicating or reducing the intensity and duration of phantom limb pain. (67)•
Urinary System	**Difficult urination**, Men above the age of 55 suffering from frequent, urgent, difficult and nocturnal urination: "(A) 10 were cured, all symptoms disappeared, (B) 5 showed markedly effective, main symptoms disappeared, (C) 30 were effective, symptoms alleviated and (D) 5 were ineffective, no improvement" (Hypertrophy of the prostate) (109)+ **Enuresis**, Children (7 to 11 years): No effect (52)*• **Enuresis**, Children (5 to 10 years): "A decrease in the night time amount of urine was reported by 43.8% of the parents, and 23.5% moved from the category of 'soaking wet' to 'a little wet'" (154) **Enuresis**, Children (3-12 years old with history of enuresis for 2-10 years) Good effect. (126)+ **Incontinence** in middle-aged women: Urinary incontinence reduced; Vaginal contraction improved; Daily life discomfort reduced (17)*^ **Incontinence** in middle-aged women: Significant change in the number of daytime frequency in the reflexology group. 24-hour micturition frequency in both groups, but the change was not statistically significant (36)*•
White blood cell count	*See Leukopenia*

Chapter Seven

Formula for Reflexology Dosing as Shown by Research

Key

* Controlled study
• PubMed (National Institute of Health)
^ Published in a peer-reviewed journal (Korea)
+ Published in a peer reviewed journal (China)

Formula for Reflexology Dosing as Shown by Research

Disorder	Frequency	Results
Aggression and anti-social behavior in children	Weekly for 8-15 weeks	Reduction in aggression, stress and anxiety and an improvement in focus, concentration, self esteem, listening skills and confidence (Aggressive and anti-social children / improving behavior to "mainstream" them into a regular classroom) (137)
AIDS (Pain and fatigue)	2 sessions over 4 days	Significant difference: less pain and fatigue; No significant difference on a 1-item numeric pain intensity scale (42)*
Anxiety	60 minutes	Reduced (Healthy individuals) (41)*•
	20 minutes, days 2, 3, 4 after surgery	Less anxiety and pain for cancer patients post operatively (157)*
	30 minutes, three times a week for 4 weeks	Significant decrease (Partner delivered) (Cancer) (21)*•
	1 session	Significant decrease (Cancer: second and third round of chemotherapy) (23)*•
	Twice per week for 5 weeks	Significant decrease (Coal workers' pneumoconiosis patients)(1)*^
	30 minutes	Significant decrease (Cancer) (134)•
	2 weeks education on theory; 4 weeks practical skill education, 3 weeks session	Decreased (Student nurses) (19)*^
	4-6 sessions	Relief from (Palliative care patients) (80)•
	30 minutes per day for 5 days	No significant changes (Coronary Artery Bypass Graft) (29)*•
	9 sessions over 9 weeks	"… reduced menopausal symptoms of anxiety, depression, hot flushes and night sweats by some 30%-50% of what they were at the outset…. "No significant difference between treatment and control group (foot massage)." (Menopausal women) (37)*•

Disorder	Frequency	Results
Arthritis (Shoulder/ acromioclavi- clar)	30 minutes per day for 15 days	8 were "cured;" 20 were "distinctly effective;" 14 cases were "improved" (Arthritis) (43)+
Asthma	60 minutes per week for 10 weeks	Reflexology and sham reflexology groups both showed decrease in beta-2 agonists and increase in peak-flow rates.(44)*•
	40-50 minutes daily for 2 to 12 weeks	Disappearance of symptoms (142)*
	45 minutes once a week for 10 weeks	No evidence that reflexology had a specific effect beyond a placebo influence (139)*•
Birthing / Delivery	During delivery	Effective pain killer (90% effective pain killer, 78% avoided surgery for placenta) (48)
	During labor	Effective pain killer (94% effective pain killer, 25% reduction in time for birth process) (47)*
	10 sessions	Reduced labor time (1/3 the labor time compared to control group) (46)
	4 or more sessions	Less analgesia /more forceps deliveries but no difference onset of labour / duration of labour (45)*•
	10-15 minutes daily	Lactation in new mothers started in 72 hours (96)*+
	Two sessions each of 30 minutes	When treated with reflexology, 70% of women diagnosed with primary inertia during labour made progress (165)*
Blood pressure	Daily for 30-40 days	Significant difference: Blood pressure/heart rate: reflexotherapy group (before): +185/80 / 86-74 and (after): +160/75 / 72-70; Blood pressure/heart rate: pharmacotherapy group (before): +180/80 / 78-72 and (after): +160/80 / 76-70 (Coronary heart disease patients) (30)*+
	Twice a week for 6 weeks (Foot reflexology)/ Twice a week for 4 weeks (Self foot reflexology)	Significant difference: (Hypertensive patients) (11)*•^
	Once per week for 4 weeks, 30 minutes each	Significantly greater decrease (Nursing home residents) (31)*•

Disorder	Frequency	Results
	20 minutes; 10 minutes	Decrease (Healthy volunteers) (137)
	Twice a week for 6 weeks	Decrease (Elderly with hypertension) (8)*^
	1 session	Lowered (Senior citizens) (28)•
	Real time	Lowered: Before: 146 mmHg.; After: fell to about 130 mmHg. (Healthy volunteers) (137)
	One session	No significant difference when foot reflexology compared to foot massage (Healthy individuals) (26)*
	Three times weekly, 45 minutes, 8 weeks	(Senior citizens) (25)*•
Blood pressure (Systolic)	60 minutes	Significant difference: (Healthy volunteers) (41)*•
	1 session	Significant difference: (Cancer patients/chemotherapy) (5)*^
	1 session	Significant difference (Cancer chemotherapy patients) (42)*
	Twice per week for 6 weeks	Decrease in (Elderly with hypertension) (8)*^
	30 minutes / 5 days	Lowered significantly (Coronary artery bypass patients) (29)*•
	Daily, 30 - 40 days	Lowered significantly (Coronary heart disease patients) (30)*+
	10 minutes, 5 days a week for one week	Significantly lower: (Cancer) (Hand reflexology) (152)*
	Daily for 6 weeks	Statistically significant difference: (Middle-aged women) (Self Foot Reflexology) (3)*•^
	Foot reflexology twice per week for 6 weeks; Self foot reflexology twice per week for 4 weeks	Statistically significant difference: (Hypertensive patients) (Self Foot Reflexology) (11)*•^
	Weekly for 6 weeks	Difference from control group (progressive meuscle relaxation) (Multiple sclerosis) (167)

Disorder	Frequency	Results
Blood pressure (Diastolic)	1 session	Significant difference (Cancer / chemotherapy patients) (42)*
	1 session	Significant decrease • (Cancer patients/chemotherapy) (5)*^
	Daily, 30-40 days	Significant decrease (Coronary heart disease patients) (30)*+
	Weekly for 6 weeks	Difference from control group (progressive meuscle relaxation) (Multiple sclerosis) (167)
	60 minutes	No significant difference 60 minutes (Healthy individuals) (41)*•
	Twice a week for six weeks, as well as self administered foot reflexology twice a week for four weeks.	No significant difference (Hypertension in the elderly) (8)*^
	30 minutes / 5 days	No significant changes (Coronary artery bypass patients) (29)*•
	10 minute daily for 5 days, one week	Not significantly lower (Cancer) (Hand reflexology) (152)*
	Three times per week for 45 minutes over 8 weeks	Reductions in diastolic blood pressure, systolic blood pressure pre-test to post-test (Foot reflexology mat walking) (Senior citizens) (25)*•
	Daily for 6 weeks	No statistically significant difference (Middle-aged women) (Self Foot Reflexology) (3)*•^
	Foot reflexology 2 / week for 6 weeks; Self foot reflexology 2 / week for 4 weeks	No statistically significant difference (11)*•^ (Hypertensive patients)
Cancer	30 minutes three times a week for 4 weeks	**Pain, anxiety:** Significant decrease pain/anxiety (21)*•
	30 minutes	**Pain, anxiety:** Significant decrease pain/anxiety (134)•
	Two times / 24 hours apart	**Pain:** Effective for alleviating fatigue (57)•

Disorder	Frequency	Results
	3 minute footsoak/10 minutes reflexology with jojoba oil containing lavender / 8 times	**Fatigue:** Effective for alleviating fatigue (24)•
	40 minutes	**Quality of life:** Improvement in quality of life: appearance, appetite, breathing, communication (doctors), communication (family), communication (nurses), concentration, constipation, diarrhoea, fear of future, isolation, micturition, mobility, mood, nausea, pain, sleep and tiredness. (151)•
	10 minutes	**Pain, nausea, relaxation:** Significant and immediate effect in pain, nausea and relaxation (22)•
	20-30 minutes daily	**Nausea and vomiting:** Significant improvement (158)*+ (Bamboo stepping)
	4 phases / 40 minutes / 8 weeks	**Nausea, vomiting, fatigue:** Decrease in nausea, vomiting, fatigue (4)*•^
	1 session	**Anxiety:** Decrease of 7.9 on state-anxiety versus 0.8 for control group (Cancer patients) (23)*•
	Unknown	**Chemotherapy:** Significant difference in: Systolic blood pressure, Diastolic blood pressure, Pulse rate, General fatigue, Mood status, Foot fatigue (5)*^
	• Hand reflexology • Ten minutes each time, five times during five days	**Radiotherapy (fatigue, anxiety, mood):** Significantly lower: The degree of fatigue, anxiety, and mood state; Lower: systolic blood pressure and pulse rate in the experimental group; Diastolic blood pressure in the experimental group were not significantly lower than that of the control group (152)*
	20 minutes, days 2, 3, 4 after surgery	**Pain and anxiety postoperatively:** Less anxiety and pain for cancer patients post operatively (157)*
	8 weeks	**Lowered levels of depression, anxiety, spirituality;** Increased levels of emotional quality of life and total quality of life Hand or foot reflexology, (Guided imagery, and/or reminiscence therapy) (140)

Disorder	Frequency	Results
	Weekly for 8 weeks	• No statistically significant effects for: "Endocrinological and immunological parameters (lymphocyte subsets, cytokine production, and hormones, prolactin, cortisol, growth hormone) thought to be relevant to an anti-tumour response" • Fewer B lympho-cytes • Quality of life: Statistically significant but modest (Post surgical breast cancer) (168)*
Cerebral palsy	Daily for 30 days	Significant improvements compared to control group: Reflexology group: Increase in growth quotient of 30-35 in those 3 to 9 months old and 10-15 with those from 1.5 to 3 years; Control group: Increase in growth quotient was 10-16 for 3-9 months and 9-15 for 1.5 to 3 years (Cerebral palsy) (49)*+
Cervical spondylosis (Degeneration of cervical vertebrae or pad between vertebrae)	Daily for 10 days or 20 days	Treatment group: Clinical "cure" rate, 49%; Remarkably effective or effective within Courses 1 and 2, 93% Control group: Clinical "cure" rate, 27%; Remarkably effective or effective within Courses 1 and 2, 49% (116)*+
	Daily, 30-40 minutes	Symptoms of dizziness, headache, nausea, unstable steps, sweating Clinically "cured": 34 (76%) cases, disappearance of symptoms and return to work • Effective: 9 (20%) cases, symptoms relieved and return to work • No effect: 2 cases (4%) **(122)**+
Cholesterol and triglycerides in the blood (Hyperlipimia)	30-40 minute session five or six times a week for 20 sessions	Remarkable reduction in cholesterol/ Strong effect on triglycerides (Hyperlipimia patients) (84)*
	30 to 40 minutes daily for 12 days (except Sunday)	Marked statistical difference and reduction in cholesterol and monoglyceride (Hyperlipimia patients) (86)*+
	Twice per week for 6 weeks	Statistically significant differences (total cholesterol) (Menopausal women) (12)*^

Disorder	Frequency	Results
	2 / week for 6 weeks	No statistically significant difference (triglyceride, high density lipoprotein and low density lipoprotein) (Menopausal women) (12)*^
Chronic fatigue syndrome	One or more cycles of daily treatments for 10 days	70% symptoms completely disappeared, resume normal work; 30% significantly reduce the symptoms, resume normal work.(Chronic fatigue syndrome patients) (153)
COPD (Chronic obstructive pulmonary disorder)	50 minutes once a week for 4 weeks	Patients felt they had benefited from taking part in this study, indicating that there were changes in sleeping patterns, breathing, and the ability to cope with life. There was no evident change in the patients' quality of life when assessed by the quality of life questionnaires. **(149)*•**
Circulation (foot)	5 minutes	Increase in blood flow to the foot (Stepping on wooden bead mat) (Healthy volunteers) (104)
	1 session	Improvement in blood flow rate/time/acceleration as measured by Doppler sonogram (Diabetes (Type 2))(35)*
Colic	Two weeks	Significantly effective / effective for 52%; others in the reflexology group were significantly impacted in comparison to the control group (138)
Constipation	60 minutes, six times in 60 days	Relieved symptoms (30%) (Premenstrual syndrome) (15)*^
	2 weeks education on theory; 4 weeks practical skill education, 3 weeks session	Bowel function improved (Students) (19)*^
	15 sessions	Significant difference (60) (Women 30-60)
	Daily for 10 days	Significant difference. Elderly and healthy individuals to whom reflexology was applied showed significant difference. (Elderly) (59)*+
	12 weeks	Significant difference (Parent/Carer delivered) (61)* (Children)
	6 sessions of 30 minutes each	Reflexology established for children's encopresis and chronic constipation following research results (90)*•

Disorder	Frequency	Results
Deafness (Drug toxic effects)	14 to 28 sessions of 40 minutes each	Significantly effective Treatment stopped once the patient could hear a speaking voice from a certain distance (117)+
Depression	1 per week for 4 weeks, 30 minutes each	Significantly greater decrease (Nursing home patients with dementia) (31)*•
	30 minutes, 3 times per week for 4 weeks	Significant improvement in relieving pain and depression (Osteoarthritis) (13)*^
	60 minutes twice per week for 5 weeks	Significant decrease for depression and anxiety (Pneumoconiosis) (1)*^
	30 minutes, 12 sessions	Less depression disorder (Elderly women) (39)*•+
	2 weeks education on theory; 4 weeks practical skill education, 3 weeks session	Depression states decreased (Students) (19)*^
	Daily for 6 weeks	Statistically significant difference (Self help foot reflexology) (Middle-aged women) (3)*•^
	45 minutes, 9 times over 19 weeks (once a week for six weeks followed by once a month for three months)	"... reduced menopausal symptoms of anxiety, depression, hot flushes and night sweats by some 30%-50% of what they were at the outset." (Menopausal women) (37)*•
	Weekly for 14 weeks (2 series)	Temporary relief from symptoms including anger, depression and muscle tension; Improved sleep patterns, levels of concentration and a lift in overall mood (Soldiers) (Post traumatic stress syndrome) (132)
	Unknown	Significant improvements in psychological health and levels of depression over time (Victims of community violence) (Post traumatic stress syndrome) (133)
	Once a week for 4 weeks, 30 minutes each	Significantly greater decrease in pain and depression (Nursing home residents/palliative care) (31)*•
	8 weeks	Lowered levels of depression, anxiety, spirituality; Increased levels of emotional quality of life and total quality of life (Cancer) (140)

Disorder	Frequency	Results
Diabetes (Type 2)	Daily for 30 days	Greatly reduced (fasting blood glucose levels/ platelet aggregation/ length and wet weight of the thrombus/senility symptom scores/ serum lipid peroxide (33)*•+
	Daily for 30 days	Marked improvement for 67% (senility, thrombocyte aggregation rates (TAR), the length and wet weights of thrombosis in vitro, and the serum oxidative lipids) (34)*+
	1 session	Improvement in blood flow rate of the feet /time/ acceleration as measured by Doppler sonogram (Diabetes (Type 2))(35)*
	30 minutes three times per week	Improvement in pulse/fatigue/mood / No decrease in blood sugar (7)*^
	Self help foot reflexology, 6 weeks	Improving peripheral neuropathy (especially tingling and pain) / No improvement in effect: peripheral circulation (Diabetes (Type 2)) (6)*^
Digestive system *See also Colic, Constipation. Dyspepsia, Irritable bowel*	1 session	Increase in blood flow to the intestines. (Healthy volunteers) (69)*•
Dyspepsia	30 minutes once or twice a day for two weeks	Very effective (98 or 74.2%), effective (30% 22.7%), failure (4 or 0.3%) (Dyspepsia) (83)+
Edema in pregnancy	15 minutes session	Feeling of well being followed session but swelling not reduced (148)*•
Encopresis (Fecal incontinence / Chronic constipation)	30 minutes once a week for 6 weeks	Incidence of soiling decreased and bowel motions increased. (Children) (90)*•
Enuresis, Children (7 to 11 years)	14 sessions over 4 months	No effect (52)*•

Disorder	Frequency	Results
Enuresis, Children (5 to 10 years)	30-minute treatments, twice weekly for four weeks (with a minimum of 2 days between treatments), followed by weekly treatments for seven weeks.	"A decrease in the night time amount of urine was reported by 43.8% of the parents, and 23.5% moved from the category of 'soaking wet' to 'a little wet'" (154)
Enuresis, Children (3-12 years old with history of enuresis for 2-10 years)	One course of treatment = 15 sessions daily (*Unknown number of courses of sessions*)	Good effect.(126)+
Epilepsy	Daily for 2 to 3 months	Effective for 8 of the 9 cases (91)+
Falls (control over)	3 times per week for 45 minutes over 8 weeks	Greatly improved perceptions of control over falls (Self help foot reflexology) (Senior citizens) (25)*•
Fatigue	30 minutes 3times per week	Improvement in (Diabetes type 2) (7)*^
	3 minutes footsoak/10 minutes oil/ 8 times	Effective for alleviating (fatigue) (Cancer) (24)•
	Twice per week for 6 weeks	Decrease in (Hypertension in elderly) (8)*^
	4 phases for 40 minutes over 8 weeks	Decrease in (Cancer) (4)*•^
	60 minutes twice per week for 5 weeks	Decreased significantly (Pneumoconiosis) (2)*•^
	60 minutes 6 times /60 days	Relieved symptoms (50%)(Premenstrual syndrome) (15)*^
	40 minutes, twice per week for 6 weeks	Less physical, psychological, neurosensory fatigue (Hospitalized stroke) (18)*^
	45 minutes for 3 consecutive days	Lower fatigue score (Elderly women) (16)*^
	30 minutes 2 sessions over 4 days with 2 sham sessions	Significantly less (AIDS) (42)*

Disorder	Frequency	Results
	40 minutes twice per week for 4 weeks	Scores of fatigue decreased (Female nurses) (9)*^
	Twice per week for 6 weeks	Statistically significant difference (Menopausal women) (12)*^
	40 minutes twice per week for 4 weeks	Significantly lower (Self help foot reflexology) (Female nurses) (9)*^
Free radicals	30-40 minutes daily for 10 days	Increase SOD, GP, GHtal; Decrease MDA (Healthy/various illness) (51)*+
	30-40 minutes daily for 12 days	Significant difference in SOD, GHtal, MDA (Cervical spondylosis) (50)*+
Gout	30 minutes, 7 - 10 sessions	Relieved 100% of symptoms within 7 to 10 sessions: Swollen joint, pain, difficulty in walking, blood uric acid normalized (115)*+
Headache	Unknown	81% of patients confirmed that reflexology had either "cured" (16%) or helped (65%) their symptoms. 19% were able to completely dispense with the medications they were taking before the study (92)
Heart	Single session	Significantly greater reductions in Baroreceptor reflex sensitivity (26)*
	Single session	Significantly greater reductions in: Frequency of sinus arrhythmia after reflexology and foot massage increased by 43.9% and 34.1% respectively (Healthy individuals) (26)*
	Single session	Significantly greater reductions in: ECG (fall in interval ratio) both indicate increase in relaxation (Healthy volunteers) (137)
	Daily for 30-40 days	Significant difference: Reflexotherapy group (before): slight change in T-wave and (after): improved remarkably ECG; Pharmacotherapy group (before): change in ST-T wave and (after): certain improvement (Coronary heart disease) (30)*+
	Daily for 30-40 days:	Reflexotherapy group: chest distress and angina pectoris disappeared; Pharmacotherapy group: chest distress and angina pectoris disappeared (Coronary heart disease) (30)*+

Disorder	Frequency	Results
Hemodialysis	10 minutes, five / week for five weeks	Increase in hemoglobin; Decrease in blood urea nitrogen and creatinine; Increase in lymphocyte subsets; Increases in vigor, mood, uplift, self-care (Hand reflexology) (10)*^
	10 minutes, five times over 3 days	Hemoglobin levels significantly increased; Emotional responses, vigor and mood scores were significantly increased. (40)*^
	10 minutes daily	Decrease in foot cramping common to hemodialysis patients (155)
Hepatitis B	Daily for 40 days	"Cured" of Hepatitis virus: HBsAg decreased and disappeared (118)+
Hospice	4-6 sessions of reflexology	Patients identified: relaxation, relief from tension and anxiety, feelings of comfort and improved well-being (80)•
	Weekly for 6 weeks	Reflexology did not demonstrate a cumulative effect in anxiety and depression (136)*•
Immune System	Daily for 6 weeks	Statistically significant difference in Natural Killer (NK) cells and IgG antibodies (Self-foot reflexology) (Middle aged women) (3)*•^
	10 minutes a day, five days a week for 5 weeks	NK (Natural killer) cells decreased significantly and CD8 decreased "However, no significant differences between (experimental and control) groups were found." (Hand reflexology) (Hemodialysis patients) (10)*^
	10 minutes, five times over 3 days	NK (Natural killer) cells and suppressor T cells showed decreased significantly but there were no significant differences between the (Hand reflexology) (Hemodialysis patients) (40)*
Incontinence	45 minutes daily for 3 weeks	Significant change: Number of daytime frequency; No significant difference: 24 hour micturation frequency (Middle-aged women) (36)*•
	30 minutes 3 times per week for 4 weeks	Effective (Self help foot reflexology) (Middle-aged women) (17)*^

Disorder	Frequency	Results
	30 minute sessions applied once or twice a day for 10 to 21 days.	Men above the age of 55 suffering from frequent, urgent, difficult and nocturnal urination: "(A) 10 were "cured," all symptoms disappeared, (B) 5 showed markedly effective, main symptoms disappeared, (C) 30 were effective, symptoms alleviated and (D) 5 were ineffective, no improvement" (109)+
Infertility	30-40 minute session daily	One woman became pregnant after 60 days of treatment; Two after 70 days; One after 90 days (84)*
	8 sessions over 10 weeks	"The rate of ovulation during true reflexology was 11 out of 26 (42%), and during sham reflexology it was 10 out of 22 (46%). Pregnancy rates were 4 out of 26 in the true group and 2 out of 22 in the control group." (164)*
Insomnia See also **Sleep**	60 minutes twice per week for 5 weeks	Significant decrease (Pneumoconiosis) (2)*•^
	60 minutes, 6 times in 60 days	Relieved symptoms (40%) (Premenstrual syndrome) (15)*^
	6 times over 3 weeks	Clinically important improvement in sleep quality (Insomnia) (54)
	Twice a day for 10 days	100% effective and then 88% effective five days after treatment.(87)*+
	Once a day for 10 day	88% effective and then 22% effective five days after treatment.(87)*+
Irritable bowel	30 min. sessions 6 times	Not effective (55)*•
	Mean of 6 sessions	Effective (61% lost severe symptoms; 39% lost all severe symptoms, others; Not effective 21% (56)
Kidney function	10 minutes, 5 times a week for 5 weeks	Improvement in kidney's function with an increase in: red blood cells to combat anemia concerns, natural killer cells to help fight infection, and enhances disposal of waste products (Hemodialysis patients) (Hand reflexology) (10)*^
	10 minutes, five times over 3 days	Improvement in kidney function (red cells) and in vigor and mood (Hemodialysis and cancer patients) (Hand reflexology) (40)*

Disorder	Frequency	Results
	1 session	Improvement in kidney's blood flow (Healthy volunteers) (69)*•
Kidney stones (Recovery from lithotrity)	Daily for 30 minutes	Reflexology group experienced less pain, began excretion earlier, and completed the excretion process earlier. (78)*+
Kidney stones (Pain)	15 minutes	90% experienced pain relief (74)*
Lactation in new mothers	Daily 10 to 15 minutes	Satisfactory lactation occurred earlier than control group with 98% within 72 hours. (96)*+
Lipoprotein (High density and low density cholesterol)	30-40 minute session five or six times a week	Remarkable reduction in cholesterol (Hyperlipimia patients) (84)*
	30 to 40 minutes daily for 12 days (except Sunday)	Marked statistical difference and reduction in cholesterol and monoglyceride (Hyperlipimia patients) (86)*+
	Twice per week for 6 weeks	No significant decrease (Hypertension in elderly) (8)*^
	50 minutes, twice per week for 5 weeks	No significant decrease (Hypertension) (58)*
	Twice a week for 6 weeks	No statistically significant difference (triglyceride, high density lipoprotein and low density lipoprotein) (Menopausal women) (12)*^
	Twice per week for 6 weeks (Foot reflexology); Self foot reflexology twice per week for 4 weeks	No significant decrease (Hypertension) (11)*•^
Lower back pain	Once a week for 6 weeks, 40 minutes	Reduced (93)*
	Unknown number of sessions	No significant differences on the primary outcome measures of pain "Interview data revealed that the majority of participants reported treatment led to reduction in pain, increased relaxation and an enhanced ability to cope." (Chronic lower back pain)(105)*

Disorder	Frequency	Results
Menopause	30 minutes, Daily for 60 days	Symptoms disappeared (89)*+
	Twice per week for 6 weeks	Reduced climacteric (menopause) symptoms (Menopausal women) (12)*^
	45 minutes, 9 times over 19 weeks (once a week for six weeks followed by once a month for three months)	"… reduced menopausal symptoms of anxiety, depression, hot flushes and night sweats by some 30%-50% of what they were at the outset." (Menopausal women) (37)*•
Mental health	Once a week for 8 weeks for 30 minutes	Improvement in physical aspects, ability to concentrate, communication and ability to articulate ideas more effectively; significant improvement in emotional state; increase in motivation; significant increase in confidence and self-esteem levels; reduction of medication by several (88)
Mental health (Severe and enduring)	6 foot reflexology sessions over 6 to 12 weeks	"Many of the conversations during and after the reflexology sessions appeared far more meaningful and detailed… "The conversation for the client seemed more productive in comparison to many key worker/client sessions." (150)
Mental health (Post traumatic stress syndrome)	Once a week for 14 weeks followed by once a week for 14 weeks	Positive effects wear off after 3 days: Relief from symptoms including anger, depression and muscle tension; Improved sleep patterns, levels of concentration and a lift in overall mood (Israel)(132) *Recommendation following research: reflexology work two or three times a week*
	Unknown	Significant improvements in psychological health and levels of depression over time; Changes in post-traumatic stress disorder symptom severity were not significant (Northern Ireland) (133)
Mental retardation	One to two times a week for a year	Significantly improvement in height, weight, health states; social living abilities; intellectual development (IQ change increase of 1.85 years))(95)*+
Middle-aged women	Daily self foot reflexology for 6 weeks	Statistically significant difference in: Depression, Perceived stress, Systolic blood pressure, Natural-killer cells and Ig G (antibodies) (Self foot reflexology)(3)*•^

Disorder	Frequency	Results
Migraine headache	Once a week	Frequency, duration and severity reduced for female headache sufferers (130)
	Two times a week for two or three months plus a placebo drug	Reflexology as effective as Fluarizin (drug taken by control group) (94)*
Mood	30 minutes, three per week	Effective: pulse/fatigue/mood: no decrease blood sugar (Diabetes type 2) (7)*^
	10 minutes, five per week for five weeks	Significantly increased (Hemodialysis patients) (Hand reflexology) (10)*^
	10 minutes, five times over 3 days	Significantly increased (Hand reflexology) (Hemodilaysis/cancer patients) (40)*
	50-60 minutes weekly for 14 weeks (3 times a week suggested following analysis of results)	Lift in overall mood (Post-traumatic stress disorder) (132)
Multiple sclerosis	11 weeks	Alleviated motor; sensory and urinary symptoms (98)*
	Once a week for 18 weeks	Improvement in 45% of symptoms compared to 13% in the control group (97)*
	6 weeks	State anxiety (systolic blood pressure, heart rate) values better for reflexology; Cortisol values better for reflexology; Significant difference in both therapies for systolic blood pressure but favoring progressive muscle relaxation (167)
Myopia (Adolescent)	10 minutes, 10 times over 15-30 days	Total effective rate of 83.8% (Myopia (Adolescent) (119)+
Nervous exhaustion	Daily for 7 days	Symptoms of dizziness, insomnia, memory loss, indigestion and headaches "cured" or greatly improved for 75% (Nervous exhaustion) (100)
Neurodermatitis	Daily for 10 to 30 days	Effective rate for the treated group was 46.7% very effective and 53.3% effective. (99)*+
Neuropathy	Self help foot reflexology, 6 weeks	Improving peripheral neuropathy (especially tingling and pain) / No improvement in effect: peripheral circulation (Diabetes (Type 2)) (6)*^
Osteoarthritis	30 minutes, 3/week for 4 weeks	Significant improvement in relieving pain and depression (Osteoarthritis) (13)*^

Disorder	Frequency	Results
	15 minute session	Significantly less posttest pain for groups receiving either reflexology or foot massage. Reflexology did not statistically result in less pain than massage. (144)*
Ovulation	8 sessions over 10 weeks	"The rate of ovulation during true reflexology was 11 out of 26 (42%), and during sham reflexology it was 10 out of 22 (46%). Pregnancy rates were 4 out of 26 in the true group and 2 out of 22 in the control group." (164)*
Oxygen saturation, respiration, pulse rate	3 sessions	Remarkable and effective by stimulation applied of moderate strength as opposed to low strength (Healthy individuals) (124)+
Pain	2 sessions over 4 days, 30 min., with 2 sham sessions	**AIDS**: Significantly less "but no significant difference on a 1-item numeric pain intensity scale" (42)*
	During delivery	**Birthing**: 90% effective pain killer (48)
	Applied during labor	**Birthing**: 94% effective pain killer, 33% quicker birthing (47)*
	10 minutes	**Cancer**: Significant and immediate effect (22)•
	30 minutes	**Cancer**: Significant decrease (134)•
	40 minutes	**Cancer**: Benefitted (151)•
	20 minutes, days 2, 3, 4 after surgery	**Cancer**: Less anxiety and pain for cancer patients post operatively (157)*
	30 minutes three times a week, minimum of four weeks	**Cancer**: Significant decrease (Partner delivered) (21)*•
	2 times /24 hours apart	**Cancer**: Positive immediate effect in pain reduction (57)•
	1/week for 8 weeks	**Chest pain**: Complete relief (3 of 4 participants); Reduced (73)
	1 / week for 4 weeks, 30 minutes each	**Dementia (Nursing home patients with)**: Significantly greater decrease (31)*•
	6 weeks (self-foot reflexology)	**Diabetes mellitus:** Improved peripheral neuropathy (6)*^

Disorder	Frequency	Results
	7-10 sessions, 30 minutes	**Gout**: Relieved pain completely (115)*+
	After single reflexology session	**Healthy individuals**: Significant increase in pain tolerance and pain threshold (88)
	3 session in one week	**Herniated disc**: 62.5% reported reduction in pain (72)•
	Mean of 6 sessions	**Irritable bowel syndrome**: Relieved 61% of severe symptoms including pain (56)
	15 minutes	**Kidney stones**: 90% experienced complete pain relief (for over an hour; 5 of the patients pain relieved for 4 hours (74)*
	First 48 hours after surgery	**Knee replacement surgery**: Significantly less morphine use post operatively (141)*
	Three times a week	**Knee replacement surgery**: No significant difference for medication except 48 hours post surgically (141)*
	Daily for 30 minutes	**Lithotrity**: Less pain in recovery from lithotrity (78)*+
	1/week for 6 weeks	**Lower back pain**: Reduced by a median value of 2.5 cm. with minimal change in sham group (0.2) (93)*
	Unknown number of sessions	**Lower back pain (chronic)**: No significant differences on the primary outcome measures of pain "Interview data revealed that the majority of participants reported treatment led to reduction in pain, increased relaxation and an enhanced ability to cope." (105)*
	20-40 minutes	**Miscellaneous pain sufferers**: "Healed" (18 participants; 2-3 sessions); No pain (11 participants); Effective (22 participants); Ineffective (9 participants) (76)+
	Daily for 3 days post surgery	**Open heart surgery patients**: Unpleasant symptoms score was lower than 2 control groups) (106)*
	Three times per week for 4 weeks, 30 minutes each	**Osteoarthritis**: Significant improvement in relieving pain (13)*^

Disorder	Frequency	Results
	15 minute intervention	**Osteoarthritis**: Significantly less posttest pain for groups receiving either reflexology or foot massage (144)*
	1/week for 6 weeks	**Phantom limb pain**: Highly significant difference / Effective in eradicating or reducing (Practitioner or self-help) (67) •
	60 minutes, 6/60 days	**PMS/Dysmenorrhea**: Relieved symptoms (35%)(15)*^
	3 / week for 45 minutes over 8 weeks	**Senior citizens**: Significantly reduced pain (Self help / Cobblestone mat walking) (25)*•
	Daily for 2 weeks	**Sinusitis**: 36% decrease in sinus medication including pain relievers (77)*
Peptic ulcer	Foot reflexology, stomach or duodenum reflex area, two times a day, each for 15 min. to 20 min. for four weeks	Symptoms disappeared 80 cases (97.56%), two "cured" after treatment in 78 patients (95.12%) (156)*+
Phantom limb pain	1/week for 6 weeks	Phantom limb pain: Highly significant difference / Effective in eradicating or reducing pain (Practitioner or self-help) (67)•
Pneumonia	Daily	20% better than control group for average time of treatment for the course of disease (102)+
Polycystic ovaries	19 times over 5 to 6 months	Length of menstrual cycles changed significantly (103)
Post operative	15-20 minutes	Decrease in the quantity of pain killers to less than 50% in comparison to the control group (General surgery patients)(101)*
	10-30 minutes	(Uroshesis) 65% of post operative patients could urinate within 10 minutes and another 25% within 30 minutes of reflexology treatment versus 25% and 45% of control group. (Surgery of cranium or brain) (114)+
	First, second and third days after surgery	Mean of unpleasant symptoms score was lowest (with aromatherapy) (Open heart surgery patients) (106)*
	Within 24 hours of surgery	Significantly less morphine use post operatively (Knee replacement) (141)*

Disorder	Frequency	Results
	20 minutes, days 2, 3, 4 after surgery	Less anxiety and pain for cancer patients post operatively (157)*
	Three times a week	No significant difference for medication 48 hours post surgically (Knee replacement patients) (141)*
	15 minutes for 5 days	Reflexology group: More able to void without problems, Indwelling catheter removed earlier. Foot massage group (Control): significant results in the subjective measures of well-being, pain and sleep. (Post abdominal surgery)(81)*
	A few days	Reflexology group: Various effects, some negative (occasionally trigger abdominal pain), Not recommended Foot massage control group more relaxing and positive (Post gynecological surgery) (82)*
	One session	Posttest mean score on pain of an experimental group was significantly lower; Posttest mean score of frequency pain medication taking was significantly lower than of a control group (Post prostatectomy surgery) (143)*
	Unknown	Reflexology enhances urination, stimulates bowel movements and so aids recovery. Patients who received reflexology also showed a much less need for medication than patients in the control group (107)*
Post-partum women	3 consecutive days	Significantly difference in time to first defecation for reflexology group (Women recovering from Cesarean section/Gastrointestinal function) (163)*
	Unknown	Significantly shorter voiding time for "artificial" foot reflexology group and machine foot reflexology group (Women recovering from Cesarean section/Urinary system)(159)*+
	6 hours of work (?)	Foot reflexology with traditional Chinese medicine foot bath group had a significant difference in: "appetite, lactation, exhaust, Elu volume, high end of the Palais, intervention; anxiety, depression score" (159)*+

Disorder	Frequency	Results
	6 hours of work (?)	Significant difference for foot reflexology with traditional Chinese medicine foot bath group for anxiety and depression score (160)*+
	5 / week for 2 weeks	Decrease in TG (triglycerides) levels in blood serum (14)*^
	30 minutes in the evening, 5 consecutive days	Significant imrovement in quality of sleep (170)*
Post traumatic stress syndrome	Two series of weekly for 14 weeks	Positive effects wear off after 3 days: Relief from symptoms including anger, depression and muscle tension; Improved sleep patterns, levels of concentration and a lift in overall mood (Soldiers)(132) *Recommendation following research: reflexology work two or three times a week*
	Unknown	Significant improvements in psychological health and levels of depression over time; Changes in post-traumatic stress disorder symptom severity were not significant (Victims of community violence) (133)
Premenstrual syndrome	30 minutes, 1/week for 8 weeks	Significantly greater decrease in premenstrual symptoms (Foot, hand, ear reflexology) (38)*•
	60 minutes, 6/60 days	Relieved symptoms: Fatigue (50%); Insomnia (40%); Abdominal pain (35%); Lower abdominal pain (30%); Constipation (30%) (15)*^
Prostate	13 sessions	65% of participants reported a reduction in their need to urinate; 67% reported a better bladder pressure; 80% reported reduced sexual problems; 60% reported improvement of their general condition (108)
Pulse rate	60 minutes	Significant difference • 60 minutes (Healthy individuals) (41)*•
	1 / week for 4 weeks, 30 minutes each	Significant difference 1 / week for 4 weeks, 30 minutes each (Nursing home residents) (31)*•
	1 session	Significant difference (Cancer chemotherapy patients) (42)*

Disorder	Frequency	Results
	20 minutes; 30 minutes	Decreased (Physiological measures of healthy individuals) (137)
	1 session	Lowered (Senior citizens) (28)•
	Daily, 30-40 days	Lowered (Coronary heart disease patients) (30)*+
	Real time	Lowered: Before, 62; during work on right foot, 54; after work on left foot, 50 (Healthy volunteers) (137)
	10 minutes, five times over 3 days	Decreased significantly on the 1st times, but not 5th times (Hemodialysis patients) (Hand Reflexology) (40)*
	10 minutes daily for 5 days	Lowered (Cancer) (Hand reflexology) (152)*
	Daily for 6 weeks	No statistically significant difference (Middle-aged women) (Self Foot Reflexology) (Hand reflexology) (3)*•^
Respiration	3 sessions	Oxygen saturation level increased: remarkably significant difference between moderate strength of application and low strength. Respiration rate increased: Remarkably significant difference between moderate strength of application and low strength (Healthy volunteers) (124)+
Sinusitis	Daily for 2 weeks	36% of subjects in both reflexology and irrigation groups reported decreased use of sinus medication (77)*
Sleep	40 minutes, 2/week for 4 weeks	Score of fatigue decreased. Score of sleep states increased (Nurses) (9)*^
	Twice a day for 10 days / Once a day for 10 days	100% of the twice a day group no longer had a problem sleeping compared to 91% of the once a day group. • Five days after treatment, however, the effective rate was 88% for the twice-a-day group and 22% for the once-a-day group (Insomnia) (87)*+
	6 sessions over 3 weeks	Produces a clinically important improvement in sleep quality (Insomnia) (54)

Disorder	Frequency	Results
	Daily for 10 to 30 days	Reflexology is a simple, effective, economical and lacking the side effects of drugs given the control group (fatigue, sleeplessness, gastrointestinal symptoms, with hormonal dermatitis resulting from long-term use) (Neurodermatitis) (99)*+
	3 times a week for 45 minutes for 8 weeks (Reflexology mat)	• Significantly reduced daytime sleepiness and pain (Senior citizens) (25)*•
	2 cycles of weekly for 14 weeks	Improved sleep patterns, levels of concentration and a lift in overall mood (Post traumatic stress syndrome) (132)
	12 sessions, 30 minutes per session	Improved sleep quality (Elderly women) (39)*•+
	45 minutes for 3 consecutive days	Sleep score higher. Fatigue score lower. (Elderly women) (16)*^
	60 minutes, 2/week for five weeks	Scores decreased significantly for fatigue and insomnia (Pneumoconiosis (coal workers') (2)*•^
	Daily for 15 days	Better qualities of sleep Fatigue (Athletes) (53)*+
	One 40-minute session	Improvement in sleep (Cancer) (151)•
Stroke	Twice a week for 60 weeks, 40 minutes each	Improvement in activities of daily living; Less physical, psychological and neurosensory fatigue (Stroke) (18)*^
	Once a day in first course; every other day in second course; once or twice a week in third course (Course =10 sessions; work continued for some until results were achieved)	• 28 cases (74%), symptoms relieved (able to walk independently) • 8 cases (21%) fundamentally recovered (negative Babinski) (Stroke) (125)+
Triclycerides	Foot reflexology twice a week for 6 weeks; Self foot reflexology twice a week for 4 weeks	Decrease in (Hypertension) (11)*•^
	5 times a week for 2 weeks	Decrease in (Postpartum women) (14)*^

Disorder	Frequency	Results
	30-40 minutes each 5 or 6 times a week	Strong effect (High cholesterol patients) (83)+
	Twice a week for six weeks, as well as self administered foot reflexology twice a week for four weeks.	Significantly decreased (Hypertension in the elderly) (8)*^
	Twice a week for 6 weeks	No change (Menopausal women) (12)*^
	50 minute twice week for 4 weeks	No change (Hypertension) (58)*
Urinary tract infection	Daily	Reflexology with drug therapy was better than drug therapy alone. All showed disappearance of symptoms on Day 1 or 2 as opposed to disappearance of symptoms on Day 2 or 3 for drug therapy only group. (112)*+
Urinary tract stones (Lithotrity)	Daily for 30 minutes	Excretion of fragmented calculus in 7 days: reflexology group, 30; control group:5; Fifteen days or less: reflexology group: 43; control group 22. (78)+
Urinary tract stones	3-20 sessions	"Cure rate" achieved by application: 3-5 times for three individuals; 6-8 times for eight individuals; 10-12 times for eight individuals; more than 20 times for 5 individuals. (111)+
Urination	30-minute sessions applied once or twice a day for 10 to 21 days	Men above the age of 55 suffering from frequent, urgent, difficult and nocturnal urination. "(A) 10 were cured, all symptoms disappeared, (B) 5 showed markedly effective, main symptoms disappeared, (C) 30 were effective, symptoms alleviated and (D) 5 were ineffective, no improvement" (109)+
	14 sessions over 4 months	Children (7 to 11 years) No effect Enuresis (52)*•

Disorder	Frequency	Results
	30-minute treatments, twice weekly for four weeks (with a minimum of 2 days between treatments), followed by weekly treatments for seven weeks	Children (5 to 10 years) "A decrease in the night time amount of urine was reported by 43.8% of the parents, and 23.5% moved from the category of 'soaking wet' to 'a little wet'" (Enuresis) (154)
	One course of treatment = 15 sessions daily	Children (3-12 years old with history of enuresis for 2-10 years) Good effect. (126)+
	30 minutes 3/week for 4 weeks (Self foot reflexology)	Incontinence in middle-aged women (17)*^ Urinary incontinence reduced; Vaginal contraction improved; Daily life discomfort reduced
	45-minutes daily for 3 weeks	Incontinence in middle-aged women (36)*• Significant change in the number of daytime frequency in the reflexology group. 24-hour micturition frequency in both groups, but the change was not statistically significant
White blood cell count (low)	Daily, one month to one year	Symptoms relieved: Upper respiratory tract infection, Urinary infection, Insomnia, Weakness; White blood cell count improved (121)*+

Chapter Eight

Benchmarks for Dosing and Results

Key
* Controlled study
• PubMed (National Institute of Health)
^ Published in a peer-reviewed journal (Korea)
+ Published in a peer reviewed journal (China)

Benchmarks for Dosing and Results

Frequency of reflexology work	Results of reflexology research
Real time (as reflexology technique is applied)	• Birthing: Pain killing during delivery (47)• (48) • Birthing: Shorter labor time; surgery for retention of placenta avoided (47)* (48) • Brain: Activation in the brain of area reflected by big toe (temporal lobe) and cerebellum as measured by fMRI (Healthy volunteers) (127) • Brain: Stimulation to the eye reflex area resulted activation in the brain of vision-related areas, cerebellum and primary motor area as measured by fMRI (Healthy volunteers) (128) • Brain: Stimulation to the adrenal gland reflex area resulted activation in the brain of emotional, homeostatic, pain center and sensory motor cortex as measured by fMRI (Healthy volunteers) (129) • Brain: Stimulation to the eye, shoulder and small intestine reflex areas of the foot resulted in activation in the brain of areas related to the foot and also to the areas related to the eye, shoulder and small intestine or neighboring body parts as measured by fMRI (169) • Feet: Blood flow increased to the feet as measured by Doppler sonogram before and after reflexology work (Diabetes) (35)* • Heart: Moderate improvement in heart function. Three diameters of cardiac function were compared and in "most of the cases under study due to the effect of reflexological stimulation have changed significantly" as measured by ECG during electric foot roller application to heart reflex area. (Healthy volunteers) (63) • Heart rate, blood pressure decreased; Carbon dioxide density exhaled from nose increased 9%; and ECG both indicate increase in relaxation (Healthy volunteers) (137) • Intestines: Blood flow increased to intestines as measured by Doppler sonogram before, during and after work (Healthy volunteers) (68)*• • Kidneys: Blood flow increased to kidneys as measured by Doppler sonogram before, during and after work (Healthy volunteers) (69)*• • Relaxation: Creation of brain waves indicating relaxation as measured by EEG (Healthy volunteers) (64) (65)• (66)• (137)

Frequency of reflexology work	Results of reflexology research
Single session (Results of single session application	• Anxiety: reduced; (Healthy volunteers) (41)*•; (Cancer) (21)*•; (Cancer) (23)*•; (Cancer) (134)• • Circulation of blood in feet improved: massage sandals (Volunteers) (120)+; wooden bead mat walking (Volunteers) (104) • Cortisol: No significant difference (Healthy individuals) (41)*• • Labor: 70% of women in labor with primary inertia who received 2-30 minute reflexology sessions showed progress (increased dilation of the cervix). (165)• • Melatonin: No significant difference (Healthy individuals) (41)*• • Oxygen saturation, respiratory rate increased (Healthy individuals) (124)+ • Pain threshold and tolerance: Increased (Healthy volunteers) (75) • Pain: Reduced (Post operatively, cancer) (22)• (102)+ • Pain: Reduced (Cancer) (134)• • Pain (Kidney and ureter stones): Complete pain relief (90%) for 15 minutes (lasted an hour, for some lasted 4 hours) (Kidney stones) (74)* • Pain (Surigcal ward): Significant pain relief, improvement in feeling and an increase in skin temperature Pain (Surigcal ward) (172) • Pulse rate, respiratory rate, blood pressure: Lowered (Healthy volunteers) (41)*•, (Senior citizens) (28)•, (Cancer) (5)*^ • Quality of life: Improved (Cancer) (151)• • Uroshesis (urination after surgery): Improved (Brain surgery patients) (114)+

Frequency of reflexology work	Results of reflexology research
Daily	**3 days** • Sleep score higher / Fatigue score lower (Elderly women) (16)*^ • Post surgical pain (Open heart surgery): Lowest of three groups (106)* • Post surgical pain (Cancer patients): Less pain (days 2, 3,4 after surgery) (157)* **A few days** • Post-gynecological surgery recovery: Not recommended: occasionally trigger abdominal pain; Various effects, some negative (82)* **Unknown** • Cancer (Chemotherapy): Significant reduction in nausea and vomiting (Bamboo stepping/ 3 times a day for 20-30 minutes) (158)*+ **5 days** • Systolic blood pressure; Lowered significantly (Coronary bypass patients) (29)*• • Systolic blood pressure and pulse rate: Lower (Hand reflexology) (Cancer) (152)* • Diastolic blood pressure: No significant changes (Coronary bypass patients) (29)*• • Diastolic blood pressure: Not significantly lower (Hand reflexology) (Cancer) (152)* • Degree of fatigue, anxiety, and mood state: Significantly lower (Hand reflexology) (Cancer & radiotherapy) (152)* • Post surgical recovery (Abdominal surgery) More able to void without problems; Indwelling catheter removed earlier however slept worse, more pain; Control, foot massage group: significant results in the subjective measures of well-being, pain and sleep. (81)* • Post partum women: Significant improvement in quality of sleep. (170)*

Frequency of reflexology work	Results of reflexology research
Daily	**7 days** Nervous exhaustion (chief symptoms were dizziness, insomnia, memory loss, indigestion and headaches): 40% experienced complete 'cure,' further 35% had greatly improved, and a further 15% had mildly improved. Only 10% showed no change at all to the treatment. (100) **10 days** • Chronic fatigue syndrome: 70% symptoms completely disappeared, resume normal work; 30% significantly reduce the symptoms, resume normal work. (153) • Constipation: Significant difference (Elderly) (60) • Free radicals: Improvement in measures (Healthy individuals) (51)*+ • Free radicals: Significant difference in measures of free radicals (Cervical spondylosis) (50)*+ • Insomnia: Twice a day for 10 days produced 100% effectiveness. Once a day for 10 days showed 91% effectiveness. Five days after treatment, the rates were 88% for twice a day and 22% for once a day. (86)*+ **10-21 days** • Urination (frequent and urgent nocturnal): Significantly effective or effective for 90% (Prostate (Hypertrophy)) (109)+ **10-30 days** • Neurodermatitis: Very effective 47%; Effective 53% (99)*+ **12 days** • Cholesterol: Marked statistical difference and reduction (Hyperlipimia) (85)+ **2 weeks** • Dyspepsia: Very effective for 75% (Dyspepsia patients) (83)+ • Sinusitis: 36% reported decreased use of sinus medication (Sinusitis) (77)* **15 days** • Arthritis (Shoulder/acromioclaviclar): 8 were "cured," 20 were "distinctly effective," 14 cases were "improved" (43)+ • Fatigue and muscle soreness, quicker recovery from (Athletes) (53)*+ • Sleep: Better qualities of (Athletes) (53)*+ **20 days** • Myopia, Total effective rate of 83.8% (119)+ **3 weeks** • Incontinence; Significant change (Daytime frequency) but not 24 hour frequency (Middle aged women) (36)*• **3-4 weeks** • Cholesterol: Remarkable reduction (Hyperlipimia patients) (84)* **4 weeks (Twice a day)** • Peptic ulcer: Symptoms disappeared for 97.5% (156)*+

Frequency of reflexology work	Results of reflexology research
Daily	**30 days** • Pancreas (Measures of functioning): Greatly improved (Diabetes) (33)*•+ • Pancreas (Measures of functioning): Marked improvement for 67% (Diabetes) (34)*+ • Significant improvements: Cerebral palsy (49)*+ **30-40 days** • Blood pressure, pulse rate: Significant difference (Coronary heart disease patients) (30)*+ • **ECG:** Significant difference, improved remarkably (Coronary heart disease) (30)*+ • **Pulse rate**: (before) 86-74 and (after) 76-70 (Coronary heart disease patients) (30)*+ **6 weeks** • Systolic blood pressure: Statistically significant difference (Middle aged women)(3)*•^ (Self help foot reflexology) • Depression: Statistically significant difference (Middle aged women)(3)*•^ (Self help foot reflexology) • Stress: Statistically significant difference (Middle aged women)(3)*•^ (Self help foot reflexology) • Natural killer cells and IgG (Immunoglobulin G) antibodies: Statistically significant difference (Middle aged women)(3)*•^ (Self help foot reflexology) • Cortisol: No statistically significant difference (Middle-aged women) (3)*•^ (Self-help foot reflexology) • Diastolic blood pressure: No significant changes (Coronary artery bypass patients) (29)*• **70 days** Myopia: 24 eyes fully recover; 21 eyes significantly effective (123)+ **2 to 12 weeks** • Asthma (Children ages 1-7): Clinical symptoms disappeared (45)*• **1-2 years** (Leukopenia) (Pathologically low white blood cell count): More effective than medication; Symptom free or effective for symptoms (93%) with improvements in white blood cell count (Leukopenia)(121)*+
Five times a week	**1 week** • Fatigue, anxiety, and mood state: Significantly lower (Hand reflexology) (Cancer & radiotherapy) (152)* • Blood pressure (systolic) and pulse rate: Lower (Hand reflexology) (Cancer) (152)* • Blood pressure (diastolic): Not significantly lower than that of the control group (Hand reflexology) (Cancer) (152)*

Frequency of reflexology work	Results of reflexology research
Five times a week	**2 weeks** • Triglycerides: Decrease (Postpartum women) (14)*^ **5 weeks** • Improvement in kidney's function with an increase in: red blood cells to combat anemia concerns, natural killer cells to help fight infection, and enhances disposal of waste products (Hemodialysis patients) (Hand reflexology) (10)*^ • Improvement in immune system function (Hemodialysis patients) (Hand reflexology) (10)*^ • Improvement in kidney function (red cells) (Hemodialysis and cancer patients) (Hand reflexology) (40)* • Improvement in vigor and mood (Hemodialysis and cancer patients) (Hand reflexology) (40)*
Twice in 24 hours	Pain: Positive immediate effect (No statistical difference 3 hours after or 24 hours after) Cancer (Pain) (57)•
Two sessions over 4 days	Fatigue and pain: Significantly less (AIDS) (42)*
Three times a week	**1 week** • Pain of herniated disc: 62.5% reported a reduction in pain (72)• **4 weeks** • Incontinence: Urinary incontinence reduced; Vaginal contraction improved; Daily life discomfort reduced (Middle aged women) (17)*^ (Self-help foot reflexology) • Pain: Significant improvement (Osteoarthritis) (13)*^ • Pain, anxiety: Significant decrease (Cancer) (21)*• **8 weeks** • Blood pressure (Diastolic); Pre-test to post-test (Systolic): Reduction (Senior citizens)(25)*• (Self-help foot reflexology) • Falls: Greatly improved perception of control over (Senior citizens)(25)*• (Self-help foot reflexology) • Pain: significantly reduced (Senior citizens)(25)*• (Self-help foot reflexology / Cobblestone mat walking) • Daytime sleepiness, significantly reduced (Senior citizens)(25)*• (Self-help foot reflexology) **Unknown length of time** • Improvement in fatigue (Diabetes) (7)*^ • Improvement in foot fatigue (Diabetes) (7)*^ • Improvement in mood (Diabetes) (7)*^ • Improvement in pulse rate (Diabetes)(7)*^ • Improvement in pain (Diabetes) (7)*^

Frequency of reflexology work	Results of reflexology research
Twice a week	**3 weeks** • Insomnia Produced a clinically important improvement in sleep (Insomnia) (54) **4 weeks** • Anxiety (Female nurses) (9)*^ • Bed wetting (Enuresis) A decrease in the night time amount of urine (154) • Blood pressure, No statistically significant difference (Hypertension) (58)* • Cholesterol, No statistically significant difference (Hypertension) (58)* • Diastolic Blood pressure No statistically significant difference (Hypertensive patients) (11)*•^(Self-help foot reflexology) • Fatigue state score: Increased /Improved (Female nurses) (9)*^ • Life satisfaction (Hypertensive patients) (11)*•^ • Lipoprotein No significant decrease (Hypertension)(11)*•^ (Self foot reflexology) • Sleep states score: Increased/ Improved (Female nurses) (9)*^ • Systolic blood pressure: Decrease (Hypertensive patients) (11)*•^ • Triclycerides: No statistically significant difference (Hypertension) (58)* **5 weeks** • Anxiety: Significant difference (Coal workers' pneumoconiosis patients) (1)*^ • Depression: Significant decrease (Coal workers' pneumoconiosis patients) (1)*^ • Fatigue: Significant decrease (Coal workers' pneumoconiosis patients)(2)*•^ • Insomnia: Significant decrease (Coal workers' pneumoconiosis patients)(2)*•^ **6 weeks** • Blood pressure (Systolic and diastolic): Decrease (Elderly with hypertension)(8)*^ • Blood pressure (Systolic): Decrease (Hypertensive patients) (11)*•^ • Blood pressure (Diastolic): No statistically significant difference (Middle-aged women) (3)*•^ • Blood pressure (Diastolic): No statistically significant difference (Hypertensive patients) (11)*•^ • Cholesterol (total): Reduced, (Menopausal women) (12)*^ • Cortisol: Reduced (Menopausal women) (12)*^ • Fatigue: Decrease in (Hypertension in elderly) (8)*^ • Fatigue: Reduced (Menopausal women) (12)*^ • Fatigue (Physical, psychological, neurosensory) (Hospitalized stroke) (18)*^ • Lipoprotein No significant decrease (Hypertension) (11)*•^ • Lipoprotein No significant decrease (Hypertension in elderly) (8)*^

Frequency of reflexology work	Results of reflexology research
Twice a week	• Menopause symptoms, reduced (Menopausal women) (12)*^ • Thyroid: Significantly improved symptoms; No change in thyroid hormones (172) • Triclycerides: Decrease (Hypertensive patients) (11)*•^

Frequency of reflexology work	Results of reflexology research
Once a week	**4 weeks** • Pain reduction: Significantly greater decrease (Nursing home patients with dementia) (31)*• • Alpha amyase: Significantly greater decrease (Nursing home patients with dementia) (31)*• • Blood pressure: Significantly greater decrease (Nursing home patients with dementia) (31)*• • Cortisol: Significantly greater decrease (Nursing home patients with dementia) (31)*• • Depression: Significantly greater decrease (Nursing home patients with dementia) (31)*• • DHEA: Significantly greater decrease (Nursing home patients with dementia) (31)*• • Heart rate: Significantly greater decrease (Nursing home patients with dementia) (31)*• **6 weeks** • Encopresis (Fecal incontinence) / Constipation in children (90)*• Results so successful that reflexology was established as method of care (90)*• • Pain reduction, Significant difference/Effective in reducing or eradicating (Phantom limb) (67) • (Foot reflexology) • Pain reduction, Significant difference/Effective in reducing or eradicating (Phantom limb) (67) • (Self-help hand reflexology) • Pain reduction, VAS median of 2.5 compared to 0.2 of control group (Lower back) (93)* • Multiple sclerosis: Difference in heart rate, systolic blood pressure, cortisol (167) **8 weeks** • Pain relief: Complete/reduced (Chest pain) (73) • Mental health, Improvement in: physical aspects, emotional state, ability to concentrate, motivation for a significant number of participants, confidence and self-esteem levels, communication and ability to articulate ideas more effectively (Mental health) (88) • PMS, significantly greater reduction in symptoms (38)*• • Endocrinological and immunological parameters (prolactin, cortisol, human growth hormone, T lymphocyte subsets or cytokine production) thought to be relevant to an anti-tumour response: No statistically significant effects. Fewer B lympho-cytes. Statistically signifcant but modest effects on quality of life. (Post surgical breast cancer patients) (168)*

Frequency of reflexology work	Results of reflexology research
Once a week	**8 to 15 weeks** • **Children:** Reduction in aggression, stress and anxiety and an improvement in focus, concentration, self esteem, listening skills and confidence. (Aggressive, anti-social behavior in children / Mainstreaming) (135) **10 weeks** • Asthma: No evidence of a specific effect on asthma beyond a placebo influence (139)*• **11 weeks** • Multiple sclerosis: alleviated motor: sensory and urinary symptoms in MS patients (98)* **14 weeks** • Post traumatic stress syndrome: Temporary relief from symptoms including anger, depression and muscle tension; Improved sleep patterns, levels of concentration and a lift in overall mood. Relief provided for 3 days. Researchers suggest work 2 or 3 times per week. (132) **18 weeks** • Multiple sclerosis: 45% improvement of symptoms compared to 13% in control group (97)* **One year** • Mental retardation: Improvement in height, weight, health states, social living abilities, intellectual development (1.85 years) (95)*+ **Unknown** • Migraine headache: Reduced frequency, duration and severity (130)
15 sessions	Constipation: Significant difference (Women 30-60) (60)
13 sessions	Prostate (men of age 55): Urination: 65% reported a reduction in their need to urinate; Bladder pressure: 67% reported a better bladder pressure; Sexual problems: 80% reported reduced sexual problems; General condition: 60% reported improvement of their general condition (Prostate) (108)
2 weeks	Colic: Significant difference (Colic) (138)
12 weeks	Constipation: Significant difference (Parent/carer delivered) (Children) (61)*
12 sessions	• Depression: Less depressive disorder (Elderly women) (39)*•+ • Serotonin: Higher level than control group (Elderly women) (39)*•+ • Sleep: Improved sleep quality (Elderly women) (39)*•+
11 weeks	Multiple sclerosis: Specific reflexology treatment was of benefit in alleviating motor; sensory and urinary symptoms in MS patients. (98)*

Frequency of reflexology work	Results of reflexology research
10 sessions	Birthing (Labor outcomes): Reflexology group experienced: average first stage was 5 hours, second stage 16 minutes, and third stage 7 minutes; compared to textbook figures of 16 to 24 hours' first stage, and, 1 to 2 hour's second stage (46)
10 times over 15-30 days	Myopia (Adolescent): Total effective rate of 83.8%. After two courses of treatment among the 68 eyes:10 (14.7%) showed more than 0. 5 increase in visual acuity; 23 (33.8%) increased by 0.25-0.40; 24 (35.3%) by 0.1-0.25: 10 minutes (119)+
7-10 sessions	Gout: Relieved 100% of symptoms (Swollen joint, pain, difficulty in walking, blood uric acid normalized) (115)*+
6 sessions over 60 days	PMS/Dysmenorrhea: Relieved symptoms: Fatigue (50%); Insomnia (40%); Abdominal pain (35%); Lower abdominal pain (30%); Constipation (30%) (Students) (15)*^
4-6 sessions	Hospice: Patients identified: relaxation, relief from tension, feelings of comfort and improved well-being (80)•
6 sessions	Encopresis (Fecal incontinence)/ Constipation in children: Research results so successful that reflexology was established as method of care (90)*•
9 sessions over 19 weeks	Menopausal symptoms: "… reduced menopausal symptoms of anxiety, depression, hot flushes and night sweats by some 30%-50% of what they were at the outset." (37)*•
4 phases for 40 minutes over 8 weeks	Cancer & chemotherapy, decrease in Nausea, Vomiting, fatigue (4)*•^
8 times	Fatigue (Cancer), Effective for alleviating fatigue in terminally ill cancer patient (Cancer) (24)•
6 weeks	Neuropathy (Diabetes) Good effect: Improving peripheral neuropathy (especially tingling and pain) Not effective: Improving peripheral circulation (Self help) (Diabetes) (6)*^
4 or more sessions	Birthing (Labor outcomes) Reflexology group experienced: Less analgesia use but more forceps deliveries; No difference: onset of labour, duration of labour (45)*•
19 times over 5 or 6 months	Polycystic ovaries: Length of menstrual cycles changed significantly; Number of follicles in the ovaries showed a marginally significant average fall; Hormone Values and Quality of Life did not show statistical significant changes from before to after the treatment (103)

Chapter Nine

Formula for
Hand Reflexology,
Self Help Reflexology,
Self-Help Tool Use

Key
* Controlled study
• PubMed (National Institute of Health)
^ Published in a peer-reviewed journal (Korea)
+ Published in a peer reviewed journal (China

Formula: Hand Reflexology, Self Help Reflexology & Tool Use

Disorder	Type of Reflexology	Results and Frequency
Anxiety	Hand reflexology	Significantly lower: The degree of fatigue, anxiety and mood state. • 10 minutes daily for 5 days (Cancer patients recovering from radiotherapy) (152)*
Cancer	Hand reflexology	Significantly lower: The degree of fatigue, anxiety; Improves mood state; Lower: systolic blood pressure and pulse rate in the experimental group; Diastolic blood pressure in the experimental group were not significantly lower than that of the control group • 10 minutes daily for 5 days (152)*
Cancer	Bamboo stepping	Significantly lower nausea and vomiting • Three times daily for 20-30 minutes (158)*+
Cervical spondylosis (Degeneration of cervical vertebrae or pad between vertebrae)	Hand reflexology and tui-na group	Clinical "cure" rate, 49%; Remarkably effective or effective within Courses 1 and 2, 93%; Control group: Clinical "cure" rate, 27%; Remarkably effective or effective within Courses 1 and 2, 49% • 20-30 minute session Daily for 7 days (Course 1) and then every other day for 7 session (Course 2) to 14 sessions (Course 3) (Cervical spondylosis patients) (116)*+
Circulation (Foot)	Massage sandals	Foot blood circulation measured by laser tissue scanning equipment (120)+
Circulation (Foot), Temperature	Stepping on wooden bead mat	5 minutes; Circulation improved and temperature of the foot improved and evened out (104)
Depression	Self help foot reflexology	**Statistically significant difference:** • Daily for 6 weeks (Middle-aged women) (3)*•^
Diabetes (Type 2	Self help foot reflexology	**Improvement in peripheral neuropathy / No improvement in effect: peripheral circulation** • 6 weeks (6)*^
Falls (control over)	Self help foot reflexology	**Greatly improved perceptions of control over falls:** • 3 times per week for 45 minutes over 8 weeks/ daytime sleepiness (Senior citizens) (25)*•

Disorder	Type of Reflexology	Results and Frequency
Fatigue	Self help foot reflexology	**Effective:** • 30 minutes 3 times per week for 4 weeks (Middle-aged women) (17)*^ **Significantly lower:** • 40 minutes twice per week for 4 weeks (Female nurses) (9)*^
	Hand reflexology	Significantly lower: The degree of fatigue, anxiety; Improves mood state • 10 minutes daily for 5 days (Cancer) (152)*
Heart rate variability (ECG)	Electric foot roller (20 minutes)	Significant change due to the effect of reflexological stimulation; Measurement by ECG showed a moderate improvement of cardiac function of the heart's activity(63)+
Hemodialysis	Hand reflexology	• Increase in Hb (hemoglobin; Decrease in BUN (blood urea nitrogen) and Cr. (creatinine), Measures of the kidney function of waste removal; Significant increases in hemoglobin, Anemia (blood low in red blood cells) is common in people with kidney disease; Increase in lymphocyte subsets; CD32, CD33, CD34;CD4 increased significantly, A defective immune response leading to an increased susceptibility to infections is common in hemodialysis patients as well; Increases in vigor, mood, uplift, self-care • 10 minutes, five / week for five weeks **(10)***^
Hemodialysis and Cancer: physiological, emotional responses and immunity responses of the patients with chronic illness	Hand reflexology	• BT decreased significantly on both of the 1st and the 5th application; PR and BP were decreased significantly on the 1st times, but not 5th times; Hb (hemoglobin) levels significantly increased; Emotional responses, vigor and mood scores were significantly increased; B cell and CD19 were increased significantly;10 minutes, five times over 3 days (Hemodialysis and cancer patients) (40)*

Disorder	Type of Reflexology	Results and Frequency
Hemodialysis (HD) and Cramping (Common to HD patients)	Self foot reflexology	• Cramp incidences were decreased from 7.8 to 2.8 during HD and from 10.6 to 5.4 at "interdialytic period after implementation of reflexology" Reflexology applied in 11 of the total 19 incidences of cramp during HD, six incidences (54.5%) were relieved while five (45.5%) were not 10 minutes daily (66% compliance rate) **(155)**
Immune System (Depression, Stress Responses and Immune Functions of Middle Aged Women)	Self foot reflexology	Significant differences in depression, perceived stress, systolic blood pressure, natural-killer cells and Ig G • Daily for 6 weeks (3)(Middle-aged women) *•^
Lipoprotein (High density and low density)	Self help foot reflexology	**No significant decrease:** • Foot reflexology twice per week for 6 weeks; Self foot reflexology twice per week for 4 weeks (Hypertension) (11)*•^
Mood	Hand reflexology	**Significantly increased:** • 10 minutes, five times over 3 days (Hemodilaysis/cancer patients) (40)* • 10 minutes, five per week for five weeks (Hemodialysis patients) (10)*^ • 10 minutes daily for 5 days (Cancer)(152)*
Oxygen saturation, Pulse rate, Respiratory rate	Hand reflexology and foot reflexology	Remarkable and significant results produced by stimulation applied of moderate strength as opposed to low strength; Oxygen saturation rate for moderate strength: 20.50 and for low strength: 17.17; Respiratory rate for moderate strength: 98.73 and for low strength: 97.50 • 3 times, applied one hour after meals; testing conducted 1/2 hour after reflexology work (Strength of stimulus) (124)+
Pain	Self help hand reflexology	**Highly significant difference / Effective in eradicating or reducing:** • 6 weekly (Phantom limb) (67) •

Disorder	Type of Reflexology	Results and Frequency
	Self help foot reflexology	**Significantly reduced pain** • 3 / week for 45 minutes over 8 weeks (Senior citizens) (25)*• **Good effect:** • 6 weeks (Diabetes mellitus (type 2) (Peripheral neuropathy) (6)*^ **36 percent reported decreased use of sinus medication** • Daily for 2 weeks (Sinusitis) (77)*
	Hand reflexology	**Significant pain relief, improvement in feeling, an increase in skin temperature** • 5 minutes per hand (Post surgical hospital patients) (172)
Premenstrual syndrome	Foot, hand, ear reflexology	Significantly greater decrease in premenstrual symptoms • 30 minutes, once a week for 8 weeks **(38)*•**
Sleep	Self help foot reflexology	**Scores of sleep state increased:** • 40 minutes twice per week for 4 weeks (9)*^ (Female nurses) **Significantly reduced daytime sleepiness** • three times per week for 45 minutes over 8 weeks (Senior citizens) (25)*•
Stress (Sleep, Aches & pains, Mood)	Bamboo stepping (included in a program of stretching, exercise and use of massage ball)	Blood pressure normalized (reduced for those with high blood pressure; increased for those with low blood pressure) Feelings of exhaustion and malaise changed to feeling good or exhilaration Relief from pain and health problems such as constipation and insomnia (Mothers of hospitalized children, performed in the hospital) • Unknown (166)

Chapter Ten

Discussion of Negative Outcomes

Summary

Negative Outcomes
Asthma (Den)(139)*•; Asthma (Den) (142)*), Diagnosis (UK) (146); Diagnosis (Nor) (145)•; Ear disorders (Den) (Kjoller); Enuresis* (Den) (52)*•; Hospice (UK) (136)*•; Hypertension* (Australia) (58)*; Irritable bowel syndrome (UK) (55)*•; Post-surgical recovery (Austria) (82)*; Ovulation (UK) (164)*

Positive and Negative Outcomes
AIDS (42)* (Thailand); Anxiety (cortisol/melatonin) (UK) (41)*•; Birthing/Labor outcomes (45)*• (Ireland); Cancer (Post surgical breast cancer) (168)*; Cancer (Pain) (US) (57)•; Coronary artery bypass graft surgery (Anxiety) (Iceland) (29)*•; Diabetes mellitus (type 2) (Circulation) (6)*^*; Diabetes (Stress response /glucose level) (Korea) (7)*^; Diagnosis (Israel) (147); Edema (Australia) (148)*•; Hemodialysis (Korea) (10)*^; Hemodialysis (Korea) (40)*; Hypertension (Korea) (11)*•^; Hypertension in the elderly (Korea) (8)*^; Incontinence (Hong Kong) (36)*•; Lower back pain (Chronic) (UK) (105)*; Menopausal women (Korea) (12)*^; Menopause (UK) (37)*•; Middle-aged women (Korea) (3)*•; Osteoarthritis (US) (144)*; Post-surgical recovery (Austria) (81)*; Post surgical (Knee replacement) (Pain and recovery) (UK)(141)*; Post-traumatic stress disorder (Northern Ireland) (133)

Key
* Controlled study
• PubMed (National Institute of Health)
^ Published in a peer-reviewed journal (Korea)
+ Published in a peer reviewed journal (China)

Discussion of Negative Outcomes

Negative Outcomes and Protocol Issues

Asthma (44)*• (Denmark)

In a controlled study, one group received foot zone therapy and the other merely uniform clinical care but without "placebo foot zone therapy". "The 'active' group received a total of ten foot zone therapy sessions of one hour at intervals of one week. The asthmatic symptoms, consumption of medicine and the objective pulmonary function parameters were followed-up during the subsequent six months. Decrease in consumption of beta-2-agonists and increase in peak-flow levels were observed in the group which had received foot zone therapy, but the same changes were observed in the control group. The authors do not find that this investigation demonstrates that foot zone therapy is of effect on the disease bronchial asthma. They conclude, however, that the favorable effect in both of the groups are due to increased care and control which occurred in both patient groups."
Question about protocol design: Was the frequency of technique application sufficient to cause a change in symptoms?
Outcomes from other studies: Reflexology applied 40-50 minutes daily for 2 to 12 weeks demonstrated a disappearance of symptoms (142)*+.

Asthma (139)*• (Denmark)

10 weeks of active or simulated (placebo) reflexology were applied once a week. Results: "Objective lung function tests did not change. Subjective scores and bronchial sensitivity to histamine improved on both regimens but no differences were found in the groups receiving active or placebo reflexology However, a trend in favour of reflexology became significant when a supplementary analysis of symptom diaries was carried out. At the same time a significant pattern compatible with subconscious un-blinding was found." Discussion: "We found no evidence that reflexology has a specific effect on asthma beyond a placebo influence."
Question about protocol design: Was the frequency of technique application sufficient to cause a change in symptoms?
Outcomes from other studies: See above.

Diagnosis (145)• (Norway)

Seventy-six patients were examined by three reflexologists. Each patient and the therapist graded problems related to 13 different parts of the body. Results: "The statistical agreement may be better than pure chance, but is too low to be of any clinical significance."
Question about protocol design: Questionable goal of research. Reflexologists are actively discouraged from diagnosis by their professional code of ethics. In addition, reflexologists have not been taught or encouraged to develop such skills.
Outcomes from other studies: "The reflexology method has the ability to diagnose (reliable and valid) at a systematic level only, and this is applicable only to those body systems that represent organs and regions with an exact anatomic location." (147)

Diagnosis (146) (UK)

Three reflexologists chose six medical conditions which could be detected most easily and reliably. Eighteen adults with one or two of these conditions were examined by two reflexologists, blinded to the patients' condition(s). "Generally the therapists tended to score higher than the patients thus over diagnosing problems. Despite certain limitations to the data provided by this study, the results do not suggest that reflexology are a valid method of diagnosis."
Question about protocol design *See above.*
Outcomes from other studies *See above.*

Ear disorders in children* (Kjoller)(Denmark)

"A total of 98 children (with ear disorders) who received (an unknown amount of) reflexology treatment and 57 children (with ear disorders) who received treatment by a GP were included (in the study).". Results: "According to a medical evaluation there was no difference in morbidity between children treated by a reflexologist and a General Practitioner."
Protocol: Unknown frequency and number of sessions

Enuresis (52)*• (Denmark)

"An unblinded method was used comparing a treatment group (1)*^ receiving reflexology to a non-treatment group ... reflexology given as 14 treatment sessions over a period of four months did not result in a significant fall in enuresis nocturna in children aged seven to eleven years old."
Question about protocol design: Was the frequency of technique application sufficient to cause a change in symptoms?
Outcomes from other studies:
• However, some of the same Danish researchers as above (52)*• found that "Thirty-minute treatments were administered twice weekly for four weeks (with a minimum of 2 days between treatments), followed by weekly treatments for seven weeks. ... (showed) A decrease in the night time amount of urine was reported by 43.8% of the parents, and 23.5% moved from the category of "soaking wet" to "a little wet." (154)
• "It is reported that "good effect" resulted from foot reflexology treatment of 38 children with enuresis (over a regimen of daily for 15 days)" (126)+

Hospice (Cancer patients) (UK) (136)*•

"All subjects received either foot reflexology or foot massage without pressing specific areas of the feet, once a week for six weeks by three trained reflexologists. ... The results showed that there was no significant difference in the Hospital Anxiety and Depression score between the two groups. However, the symptom score showed a significant improvement in appetite and mobility for the foot massage group." Reflexology was enjoyed by the patients.
Questions about protocol design: Was the frequency of technique application sufficient to cause a change in symptoms?: The same practitioners provided both reflexology and foot massage work.
Outcomes from other studies (Hospice): "Respondents noted that their quality of life was improved through a reduction in physical and emotional symptoms. It was found that the provision of reflexology within Scottish hospices varied, with less than half providing this service. The results of this audit suggest that reflexology may be a worthwhile treatment for other cancer patients and requires further research to evaluate the benefits." (Milligan) *Continued next page*

Continued from previous page

"Patients' comments about the therapy and the service as a whole were overwhelmingly positive. They identified relaxation, relief from tension and anxiety, feelings of comfort and improved well-being as beneficial effects of their course of reflexology." (80)•

Outcomes from other studies (Anxiety): Nine studies show reduction, decrease or significant decrease in anxiety:

• Foot reflexology applied for 30 minutes; on a subsequent day, a 30-minute no intervention period was used as the control. Significantly less anxiety (Cancer) (134)•

• One-hour session. Reflexology has a "powerful anxiety-reduction effect" (state) as shown by cardiovascular parameters (BP and pulse rate) but no significant effect on underlying anxiety (trait) (cortisol and melatonin (Healthy individuals) (41)*•

• 30 minutes. Significant decrease in pain intensity and anxiety. (Cancer) (21)*•

• 1 session. Significant decrease (Cancer) (23)*•

• Significant decrease Twice per week for 5 weeks (coal workers' pneumoconiosis patients) (Coal workers pneumoconosis)(1)*^;

• Decreased. 2 weeks education on theory; 4 weeks practical skill education, 3 weeks session (Student nurses) (19)*^;

• Relief from anxiety 4-6 sessions (Palliative care patients) (80)•

• Significantly lower: The degree of anxiety. 10 minutes daily for 5 days (Hand reflexology) (Cancer)(152)*

Outcomes from other studies (Appetite)

• "100% of the reflexology group who received a 40-minute session benefited from an improvement in quality of life: appearance, appetite, breathing, communication (doctors), communication (family), communication (nurses), concentration, constipation, diarrhoea, fear of future, isolation, micturition, mobility, mood, nausea, pain, sleep and tiredness." (Cancer) (151)•

Hypertension (58)* (Thailand)

Hypertension patients The treatment group received foot reflexology 50 min. twice a week for 4 weeks. The control group received a 30-minute light foot massage session without pressure on specific reflexology areas twice a week for four weeks. "Patients receiving reflexology were compared with patients receiving a light foot massage, thus controlling for any effects contributed by massage or touch alone."

For both the unadjusted and adjusted analyses, there was no statistically significant difference between treatment groups post-intervention.... "The results from this study did not support the claim that foot reflexology can decrease blood pressure, LDL cholesterol and triglyceride levels. Similarly, there was no evidence that it could improve the quality of life in patients with hypertension.

Question about protocol design: Was the frequency of technique application sufficient to cause a change in symptoms? (B) Is foot massage appropriate as a control group? (C) Reporting of results: It was reported that there was no difference between treatment and control groups. Was there a reduction in measures using reflexology? It is not reported. There is no indication of a pretest/post-test measurement to test possible reduction in measures by either intervention. Abstract notes that "... there was no statistically significant difference between treatment groups post-intervention."

Continued on next page

Continued from previous page
Outcomes from other studies: Remarkable reduction in cholesterol and strong effect on triclycerides with a 30-40 minutes session five or six times a week for 20 sessions (Hyperlipimia patients) (84)*+
• Marked statistical difference and reduction in cholesterol and monglyceride with a 30 to 40 minute session daily for 12 days (except Sunday) (Hyperlipimia patients) (86)*+
• Statistically significant difference (total cholesterol) for twice a week sessions for 6 weeks. No statistically significant difference in triclyceride, high density lipoportein and low density lipoprotein. (Menopausal women) (12)*^
• Decrease in triclycerides five sessions per week for 2 weeks. (Post partum women) (140)•

Irritable bowel syndrome (UK) (55)*•

Six 30-minutes foot reflexology sessions were applied to 17 irritable bowel syndrome patients while the control group of 17 saw health workers with no reflexology work for 30 minutes over 6 session. "On none of the three symptoms monitored--abdominal pain, constipation/diarrhoea, and abdominal distention--was there a statistically or clinically significant difference between reflexology and control groups.".
Principle researcher Tovey notes: "I want to conclude with a note of caution. Although the results of this study are quite clear, they should not be used to dismiss reflexology as a treatment option across the board, nor indeed to argue against the effectiveness of CAM as a whole. The simple fact is that we know very little about the effectiveness of very many treatment options in relation to very many conditions. Reflexology in particular remains not just under-researched but almost unresearched — something that is quite startling given the extent of its use. For instance, we need to examine the varying impact of individual practitioners and indeed the extent to which the legitimacy held by orthodox practitioners, for instance general practitioners and/or nurses, might impinge on the effectiveness of reflexology. And even with IBS, as noted above, varying the definition and selection of patients may yet yield different outcomes. There is clearly a need for substantially more research, using a range of controlled and naturalistic approaches, before definitive conclusions can be reached."
Question about protocol design: Was the frequency of technique application sufficient to cause a change in symptoms?
Outcomes from other studies: In another study of IBS (56): Following 6 reflexology sessions and a month without treatment patient's ratings showed that: "Reflexology had little effect on the mild symptoms but the effect on severe symptoms was significant. The reductions varied from 72% to 29%. ... The variations in the effectiveness of treatment on clients' severe symptoms was related to their age, temperament and length of time with IBS."

Ovulation (England) (164)*

26 women received genuine foot reflexology and 22 received sham reflexology with gentle massage over 10 weeks. "The rate of ovulation during true reflexology was 11 out of 26 (42%), and during sham reflexology it was 10 out of 22 (46%). Pregnancy rates were 4 out of 26 in the true group and 2 out of 22 in the control group."
Question about protocol design: Was the frequency of technique application sufficient to cause a change in symptoms? Unknown if reflexology and sham reflexology were provided by the same practitioner.

Post surgical recovery (Austria) (82)*

In a study of post surgical recovery, foot reflexology or foot massage as a control or person conversation as a control applied for a few days. "The following parameters were recorded: the subjective, self-assessed, general condition, pain intensity, movement of the bowels, micturition and sleep beginning on the day before the operation until day 10."

Results: "Foot reflexology is not recommended for acute, abdominal postsurgical situations in gynecology because it has various effects, some negative, i. e. can occasionally trigger abdominal pain. Foot massage control group more relaxing and positive."

Question about protocol design: The level of pressure applied during reflexology work is unknown. Further research could determine the outcome for a lighter intensity of pressure or a generally applied reflexology technique not directed at or even avoiding foot reflex areas reflecting site of surgery.

Outcomes from other studies: Studies on reflexology applied to post-operative pain show pain reduction: "
- Patients who received foot reflexology treatment required 25 to 35 percent less standard pain medication compared to the control group" (101)* (General surgery)
- "The posttest mean score of pain of an experimental group was significantly lower than of a control group ... The posttest mean score of frequency pain medication taking of an experimental group was significantly lower than of a control group"(143)* (Elderly, prostatecy).
- The "unpleasant symptoms score" was lowest for the foot reflexology with aroma therapy group. (106)* (Open-heart surgery)

Mixed Outcomes (Positive and Negative)

AIDS (Thailand)(42)*

Foot reflexology was applied in a cross over design for 30 minutes, 2 reflexology and 2 sham sessions over 4 days. Results: Significant difference with less pain and fatigue but no significant difference on a 1-item numeric pain intensity scale.

Question about protocol design: Was the frequency of technique application sufficient to cause a change in symptoms?

Outcomes from other studies
- One study with foot reflexology applied two times 24 hours apart for 30 minutes"... found that pain scores were lowered by 2.4 points on a 0-10 pain scale in the treatment group compared to the control group immediately post intervention (n = 36, $F[1,31] = 9.08$, $p < 0.01$)" (57)• (Cancer patients)
- Application of reflexology 30 minutes three times a week, minimum of four weeks resulted in: "For the total group, 19% of the experimental group and 11% of the control group experienced pain reduction of two or more scale points on the 10-point pain scale. The intervention effect was maintained when comparing pain change scores for the moderate to severe pain subgroups, with the intervention group experiencing a 37% reduction, compared to a 6% reduction in the control subgroup. In the moderate to severe pain subgroups, 50% of the experimental subgroup and 20% of the control subgroup experienced pain reduction of two or more scale points on the 10-point pain scale." (21)*• (Cancer patients)

Anxiety, Cortisol and melatonin: (UK) (41)*•

60 minutes of "gentle" reflexology work was applied to healthy individuals.

Results: Reflexology work had a "powerful anxiety-reduction effect" and "reduced 'state' anxiety and cardiovascular activity (significant difference in: systolic blood pressure and pulse rate) within healthy individuals, consistent with stress-reduction." No significant difference was found in diastolic blood pressure. Baseline salivary cortisol and melatonin did not change significantly following reflexology.

(No other studies have measured melatonin in response to reflexology work.)

Question about protocol design (Cortisol): Frequency appears to make a difference for changes in cortisol. McVicar et. al. note this concern: "Trait anxiety, on the other hand was not significantly affected by the reflexology ... This is an expected result since trait anxiety, unlike state (anxiety as measured by systolic blood pressure and pulse rate), is not a transitory state and any changes in trait anxiety would not be expected in the time-course of this study (one session)." (41)*• "Gentle" reflexology work was utilized in this study. Would the application of "moderate" reflexology, especially to healthy individuals, make a difference in outcomes for a one-time reflexology application?

Outcomes from other studies (Cortisol): Other studies have shown a positive outcome with reflexology work:

- "significantly greater decrease" in cortisol when reflexology work was applied in 30 minute sessions once a week for 6 weeks to nursing homes residents (31)*•
- "Statistically significant difference" in cortisol when reflexology work was applied to menopausal women twice a week for 6 weeks. (12)*^
- No statistically significant difference (cortisol) when self-reflexology was applied daily for 6 weeks (Middle-aged women) (3)*•^

Question about protocol design (Diastolic blood pressure): Frequency may make a difference for changes in diastolic blood pressure as shown by other studies.

Outcomes from other studies (Diastolic blood pressure):

- Significant difference in: Pre-test/Post-test; DBP (p=.014) (Cancer / chemotherapy patients) (4)*•^; 1 session (Cancer patients/chemotherapy)(5)*^
- Significant difference in: Daily for 30-40 days; 185/80 before and 160/75 after reflexology: (Coronary heart disease patients) (30)*+;
- Decrease in: twice a week for 6 weeks (Elderly with hypertension)(8)*^;
- Reductions in: 3 / week for 45 minutes over 8 weeks (Self foot reflexology) (Senior citizens) (25)*•
- No significant changes: 30 minutes over 5 days (Coronary artery bypass patients) (29)*•;
- No significant changes: Twice a week for 6 weeks and self help twice a week for 4 weeks (Hypertension) (58)*
- Not significantly lower: 10 minute daily for 5 days, one week (Cancer) (Hand reflexology) (152)*

Anxiety (Post operative)(Iceland)(29)*•

Foot reflexology applied to coronary bypass patients for 30 minutes per day for 5 days did not reduce anxiety but did reduce systolic blood pressure.

Outcomes from other studies: Nine studies show reduction, decrease or significant decrease in anxiety:
• Foot reflexology applied for 30 minutes; on a subsequent day, a 30-minute no intervention period was used as the control. Significantly less anxiety (134)• (Cancer);
• One-hour session. Reflexology has a "powerful anxiety-reduction effect" (state) as shown by cardiovascular parameters (BP and pulse rate) but no significant effect on underlying anxiety (trait) (cortisol and melatonin (41)*• (Healthy individuals);
• 30 minutes. Significant decrease in pain intensity and anxiety. (21)*• (Cancer);
• 1 session. Significant decrease (Cancer) (23)*•;
• Significant decrease Twice per week for 5 weeks (coal workers' pneumoconiosis patients) (1)*^ (Coal workers pneumoconosis);
• Decreased. 2 weeks education on theory; 4 weeks practical skill education, 3 weeks session (Student nurses) (19)*^;
• Relief from anxiety 4-6 sessions (Palliative care patients) (80)•
• Significantly lower: The degree of anxiety. 10 minutes daily for 5 days (Hand reflexology) (Cancer)(152)*

Birthing / Delivery (Labor outcomes)(Ireland)(45)*•

Some pregnant women received 4 or more sessions. Results: Reflexology group experienced: less analgesia use and more forceps deliveries. There was no difference in onset of labour and duration of labour

Question about protocol design: Would frequency during pregnancy or during labor produce improved outcomes? It is noted at one web site that: "The findings should not be taken as particularly significant clinical value since some of the women received only one session of reflexology at 39 weeks.") (http://www.expectancy.co.uk/docs/expectancyreview.pdf)

Outcomes from other studies: Reflexology applied during the labor (47)*showed average birth process of 2.48 ± 1.48 hours compared to control group (average birth process of 3.32 ± 1.19 hours).
• Reflexology applied 10 sessions from 20 weeks on (46) showed average first stage was 5 hours, second stage 16 minutes, and third stage 7 minutes compared to textbook figures of 16 to 24 hours' first stage, and, 1 to 2 hour's second stage.

Middle-aged women (Depression, stress responses, immune system, self-help foot reflexology) (Korea)(3)*•^

Reflexology work was taught over 2 weeks of training followed by daily self foot reflexology for 6 weeks (2 days at the research center, 5 days at home) Significant difference in depression, perceived stress, systolic blood pressure, natural-killer cells and Ig G; No significant difference in diastolic blood pressure, pulse or serum cortisol.

Question about protocol design: Practitioner applied reflexology is generally believed to be more relaxing than self-help reflexology. Would results for cortisol be different with practitioner-applied reflexology?

Outcomes from other studies (Pulse): Significant difference in pulse rate, respiratory rate, blood

Continued on next page

Continued from previous page

pressure in one session (41)*• (Healthy volunteers), (28)• (Senior citizens), (5)*^ (Cancer); Daily for 30-40 days Blood pressure, pulse rate, significant difference (30)*+ (Coronary heart disease patients); Daily for 30-40 days Pulse rate: reflexotherapy group (before): pulse rate 86-74 and (after): 76-70 (30)*+ (Coronary heart disease patients); Unknown length of time Improvement in pulse rate (7)*^ (Diabetes); Significant difference for work 1 / week for 4 weeks, 30 minutes each (31)*• (Nursing home residents)

Outcomes from other studies (Diastolic blood pressure) *See above Anxiety, Cortisol, Mealtonin.*

Outcomes from other studies (Cortisol) *See above Anxiety, Cortisol, Melatonin.*

Cancer (Post surgical breast cancer) (168)*

No statistically significant effect on endocrinological and immunological parameters thought to be relevant to an anti-tumour response (prolactin, cortisol, human growth hormone) or T lymphocyte subsets, cytokine production. Fewer B lympho-cytes. Statistically significant, but modest, effects on Quality of Life.

Protocol: Who applied reflexology technique? Trained reflexologist? Same individual as applied Indian head massage? Did the timing of the interventions and testing play a role in results?

Outcomes from other studies (Cortisol): Other studies have shown a positive outcome with reflexology work:
- "Significantly greater decrease" in cortisol when reflexology work was applied in 30 minute sessions once a week for 6 weeks to nursing homes residents (31)*•
- "Statistically significant difference" in cortisol when reflexology work was applied to menopausal women twice a week for 6 weeks. (12)*^
- No statistically significant difference (cortisol) when self-reflexology was applied daily for 6 weeks (Middle-aged women) (3)*•^

Cancer (Pain)(US)(57)•

Positive immediate effect in pain reduction; No statistically significant effect 3 hours after; No statistically significant effect 24 hours after (Foot reflexology two times 24 hours apart)

Comment: Provides an indication of frequency needed to provide longer lasting pain-killing effect.

Lipoproteins (Menopausal women) (Korea) (12)*^

Reflexology was applied twice a week for six weeks. There were statistically significant differences in: climacteric symptoms (menopause), fatigue, total cholesterol, cortisol. There was no significant difference in: high density lipoprotein, low density lipoprotein, and triglycerides.

Outcomes of other studies (Triglycerides): Decrease in triglycerides for reflexology work applied twice a week for 6 weeks and twice a week for 4 weeks (Hypertension) (11)*•^ and for five times per week for 2 weeks (Postpartum women) (14)*^; Strong effect for reflexology applied 30-40 minutes 5 or 6 times a week (High cholesterol patients) (84)*+

No change for reflexology work applied 50 minute twice a week for 4 weeks (Hypertension) (58)*

Outcomes of other studies (Lipoproteins): Remarkable reduction in cholesterol for reflexology work applied 30-40 minute session five or six times a week for 20 sessions (Hyperlipimia patients) (84)*+; Marked statistical difference and reduction in cholesterol and monoglyceride for reflexol-

Continued on next page

Continued from previous page
ogy work applied 30 to 40 minutes daily for 12 days (except Sunday) (Hyperlipimia patients) (86)*+; Statistically significant differences (total cholesterol) for reflexology work applied twice per week for 6 weeks (Menopausal women) (12)*^
• No significant decrease in High density lipoprotein and Low density lipoprotein for reflexology work applied twice a week for 6 weeks and 2 / week for 4 weeks (Hypertension) (11)*•^; there was no statistically significant difference between treatment groups (foot reflexology and light foot massage) post-intervention. 50 minute 2 / week for 4 weeks (Hypertension)(58)*

Chronic obstructive pulmonary disease (COPD) (149)*•

The application of foot reflexology 50 minutes once a week for 4 weeks created a short term relaxation that did not last until the next session. Researchers noted: "We cannot make any comment based on our data as to the effect of an increased frequency of treatment on the longevity of the improvement. There was no evident change in the patients' quality of life when assessed by the quality of life questionnaires, though the evaluation questionnaire does suggest that the patients felt benefits from the study. More research is needed into this areas, since any changes in the quality of life over this short period of time may not have been picked up by the quality of life questionnaires. ... Patients felt they had benefited from taking part in this study, indicating that there were changes in sleeping patterns, breathing, and the ability to cope with life. All of these are qualitative results and would need to have further quantitative results and further qualitative analysis (if possible) before an association with the reflexology can be accurately drawn."
Interpreting efficacy: "Should patient's view of efficacy be negated because 'objective' measure showed no effect? or the appropriateness od the scientific parameters questioned because they are in conflict with patients notion of efficacy?" (Chronic lower back pain) (105)**(See page 28)*

Critically ill (UK)(Bonthron)

Neither benefit nor detrimental effects could be conclusively demonstrated for reflexology work applied to patients in an ICU (intensive care unit).
"There was sporadic recording of pain and sedation scoring. Where recorded, these sometimes seemed to contradict physiological data and/or nurses' subjective observations. Because of the many factors affecting this patient group neither benefit nor detrimental effects could be conclusively demonstrated."
"The prohibition on reflexology for the critically ill appears groundless. This being so, future research in this area is now both possible and urgently required, using appropriate methodologies to establish causative links between reflexology usage and patient outcomes."

Diabetes mellitus (type 2) (7)*^

Foot reflexology was applied 30 minutes, three times a week to patients with diabetes mellitus, type 2. Improvement in: Pulse rate, general fatigue, foot fatigue and mood but no decrease of blood sugar levels.
Question about protocol design: Was the frequency of technique application sufficient to cause a change in symptoms?
Outcomes from other studies: Reflexology applied daily for 30 days showed a change in blood sugar levels in participants. (33)*•+(34)*+

Diabetes mellitus (type 2) (6)*^

Self foot reflexology was applied for 6 weeks by patients with diabetes mellitus, type 2. A good effect was shown for improving peripheral neuropathy (especially tingling and pain) and the ability to sense 10-g monofilament on the foot. Self foot reflexology was not shown to be effective for improving peripheral circulation.
Question about protocol design: Does testing need to take place immediately after reflexology work to show improvement in circulation?
Outcomes from other studies: One session of foot reflexology applied to those with Diabetes mellitus (type 2) showed an improvement in blood flow rate, time and acceleration within the feet as tested by Doppler sonagraphic before and after work.(35)*+

Diagnosis (Isreal)(147)

80 patients were examined twice by two reflexologists "The reflexology method has the ability to diagnose (reliable and valid) at a systematic level only, and this is applicable only to those body systems that represent organs and regions with an exact anatomic location.")

Edema in Pregnancy (Australia) (148)*•

15 minutes of lymphatic reflexology work was compared to relaxing reflexology work and control rest group.
Results: Wellbeing improved significantly for those in the lymphatic reflexology group but not circumference of the ankle.
Question about protocol design: Was the frequency and duration of technique application sufficient to cause a change in symptoms?

Hemodialysis (Korea) (10)*^

Hand reflexology applied 10 minutes, five times week for five weeks showed: increase in Hb (hemoglobin); decrease in BUN (blood urea nitrogen) and Cr. (creatinine; increase in lymphocyte subsets; CD32, CD33, CD34; CD4 increased significantly and increases in vigor, mood, uplift and self-care. NK (Natural killer) cells decreased significantly and CD8 decreased "However, no significant differences between (experimental and control) groups were found."
Question about protocol design: Duration and frequency of technique application will be established with further research. Or, perhaps, research will find that reflexology does not impact these parameters.

Hemodialysis and Cancer (Korea) (40)*

Hand reflexology applied 10 minutes, 10 minutes, five times over 3 days showed: BT decreased significantly on both of the 1st and the 5th application; PR and BP were decreased significantly on the 1st times, but not 5th times; Hb (hemoglobin) levels significantly increased; emotional responses, vigor and mood scores were significantly increased; B cell and CD19 were increased significantly. Suppressor T cell and NK (Natural killer) cell showed significant decrease after the program, but no significant differences between the groups.
Question about protocol design: Duration and frequency of technique application will be established with further research. Or, perhaps, research will find that reflexology does not impact these parameters.

Hypertension (Korea)(11)*•^

Foot reflexology applied twice a week for 6 weeks and self foot reflexology twice a week for 4 weeks and compared to a control group.
Results: Decrease in systolic blood pressure, triglyceride level and improved life satisfaction but no significant decrease in diastolic blood pressure, high density lipoprotein, or low density lipoprotein.
See above discussion: Negative Outcomes, Hypertension.

Hypertension in the elderly (Korea)(8)*^

Reflexology applied twice a week for 6 weeks and applied to a control group.
Results: Decrease in systolic blood pressure, diastolic blood pressure, and fatigue but no significant decrease in serum levels, high density lipoprotein, or low density lipoprotein.
See above discussion: Negative Outcomes, Hypertension.

Incontinence (Hong Kong)(36)*•

Reflexology and control (foot massage groups) received 45-minute treatments daily for three weeks. Reflexology work "us(ed) point location with specific attention on the renal tract reflexology zone." Foot massage group used "a series of techniques with overly light pressure and not stimulating the reflex zones." Different therapists were used for each group.
Results: There was significant change in the number of daytime frequency in the reflexology group when compared with the massage group. There was also a decrease in the 24-hour micturition frequency in both groups, but the change was not statistically significant. In the reflexology group, more patients believed to have received "true" reflexology. "This reflects the difficulty of blinding in trials of reflexology. Larger scale studies with a better-designed control group and an improved blinding are required to examine if reflexology is effective in improving patients' overall outcome."
Question about protocol design: Was work applied to the appropriate reflex area? Within reflexology theory, reflexology work prompts improved function of the body part reflected by targeted reflex area. The cause of incontinence can be inappropriate signals within the nervous system, specifically the brain stem. Would work targeting the brain stem reflex area produce results?
Outcomes from other studies: A study of incontinence in middle-aged women (17)*^ showed success with self-foot reflexology was applied for 30 minutes, three times a week for 4 weeks. "Frequency, amount and the situation score of urinary incontinence were reduced significantly… "These findings indicate that self-foot reflexology is an effective method for reducing urinary incontinence symptoms and daily life discomfort and for increasing pressure of vaginal contraction"
Results were achieved when the cerebral reflex area was included in work with childhood enuresis. (126)+

Knee replacement (Pain) (UK)(141)*

Light touch full reflexology work and placebo "reflexology treatment that avoided areas thought by the reflexologists to influence the healing of the knee" were compared to a control group of usual medical care following knee replacement surgery. Treatments were applied within 24 hours of surgery and three times a week thereafter. Morphine consumption in the early postoperative period was significantly less for the two reflexology groups. No difference in length of stay in the hospital or average codydramol (pain killer given after 48 hours) used and days to reach 70° knee flexion.
Question about protocol design: Would a more moderate (versus light) pressure have changed results? Would a more frequent application make a difference?

Lipoproteins (Menopausal women) (Korea) (12)*^

Reflexology was applied twice a week for six weeks. There were statistically significant differences in: climacteric symptoms (menopause), fatigue, total cholesterol, cortisol. There was no significant difference in: high density lipoprotein, low density lipoprotein, and triglycerides.
Outcomes of other studies (Triglycerides): Decrease in triglycerides for reflexology work applied twice a week for 6 weeks and twice a week for 4 weeks (Hypertension) (11)*•^ and for five times per week for 2 weeks (Postpartum women)(14)*^; Strong effect for reflexology applied 30-40 minutes 5 or 6 times a week (High cholesterol patients) (83)
No change for reflexology work applied 50 minute twice a week for 4 weeks (Hypertension) (58)*
Outcomes of other studies (Lipoproteins): "Remarkable reduction" in cholesterol when reflexology work was applied in a 30 to 40 minute session five or six times a week for 20 sessions (Hyperlipimia patients) (84)*+; Marked statistical difference and reduction in cholesterol and monoglyceride when reflexology work was applied 30 to 40 minutes daily for 12 days (except Sunday) (Hyperlipimia patients) (86)*+; Statistically significant differences (total cholesterol) when reflexology work was applied twice per week for 6 weeks (Menopausal women) (12)*^
• No significant decrease in High density lipoprotein and Low density lipoprotein when reflexology work was applied twice a week for 6 weeks and 2 / week for 4 weeks (Hypertension) (11)*•^; There was no statistically significant difference between treatment groups (foot reflexology and light foot massage) post-intervention when either was applied for 50 minutes twice week for 4 weeks (Hypertension)(58)*

Lower back pain and functioning (chronic)(UK) (105)*

Participants were randomly assigned to reflexology, relaxation or non-intervention (usual care by GP) groups. The number of sessions is unknown.
Results: "No significant differences between the groups pre and post treatment on the primary outcome measures of pain ... and functioning ..."
• The "quantitative" data suggest that reflexology is ineffective for managing Chronic Lower Back Pain, while the "qualitative" data suggest otherwise. "Interview data revealed that the majority of participants reported treatment led to reduction in pain, increased relaxation and an enhanced ability to cope."
Question about protocol design: Unable to determine the number of sessions and frequency from available information but an issue is whether or not frequency (number) of sessions and/or intensity of technique application was sufficient to impact chronic pain. *Continued on next page*

Continued from previous page
Outcomes of other studies: Another study of lower back pain (93)* showed a positive outcome with "VAS scores for pain reduced in the treatment group by a median value of 2.5 cm, with minimal change in the sham group (0.2 cm)".
• 22 studies show outcomes ranging from "reduction in" to "significant difference in" pain.

Menopause* (UK) (37)*•

The study consisted of "…nine sessions of either reflexology or nonspecific foot massage (control) by four qualified reflexologists (applying both treatments) over a period of 19 weeks (once a week for six weeks followed by once a month for three months)…" Results: "Foot reflexology was not shown to be more effective than non-specific foot massage in the treatment of psychological symptoms (anxiety and depression) occurring during menopause." "Reflexology could not be shown to be more effective than non-specific foot massage in relieving menopausal symptoms."

Questions about protocol design:

Practitioner: Both treatment and control (foot reflexology and foot massage) were provided by the same practitioners.

Although the study does cite the method of reflexology, there is a lack of definition for reflexology technique applied. It is noted that "It (the reflexology method) does not rely on force or actual physical pressure but it gives the client the element of choice in how much his or her energies are altered by the treatment." (Study author Jan Williamson at http://www.positivehealth.com/article-abstract.php?articleid=289) It is unclear what exactly was applied during the study, pressure or energy work.

Reporting of results: Above noted results infer that reflexology was not shown to be effective for physical and psychological symptoms of menopause. However in another abstract it is noted that: "Anxiety and depression scores fell in both groups to between 50% and 70% of baseline values, with a clear time effect but no significant difference between treatment and control groups. Similar changes were found for severity of hot flushes and night sweats." (Abstract of study reported at http://positivehealth.com/permit/Updates/rudwomen2.htm) Abstract posted at the official US government site (www.ncbi.nlm.nih.gov) stated "Foot reflexology was not shown to be more effective than non-specific foot massage in the treatment of psychological symptoms (anxiety and depression) occurring during menopause." with other results reported as mean scores.

Blinding: "However this study does show the problem of devising an appropriate placebo control trial of reflexology. Future studies may benefit from the lessons gained here by avoiding attempts at blinding, eliminating the complication of non-specific effects, perhaps by using a waiting group for instance." Jan Williamson (Primary author of study, Comment posted at http://positive-health.com/permit/Updates/rudwomen2.htm)

Outcomes from other studies (Menopause): Korea (12)*^ Work applied twice a week for 6 weeks "made a statistically significant difference in climateric symptoms as well as fatigue, total cholesterol but no significant difference in high density lipoprotein, low density, triclycerice.
• China (89)+ Daily for 30 minutes over 60 days: 17 (40.48%) of the women had fully recovered (symptoms disappeared, no relapse at 2 months), 20 (47.62%) had significantly recovered (symptoms disappeared, relapse at 2 months but disappeared with more treatment), 4 (9.25%) had effective results (symptoms relieved);1 had ineffective results.

Middle-aged women (Depression, stress responses, immune system, self-help foot reflexology) (Korea)(3)*•^

Reflexology work was taught over 2 weeks of training followed by daily self foot reflexology for 6 weeks (2 days at the research center, 5 days at home) Significant difference in depression, perceived stress, systolic blood pressure, natural-killer cells and Ig G; No significant difference in diastolic blood pressure, pulse or serum cortisol.

Question about protocol design: Practitioner applied reflexology is generally believed to be more relaxing than self-help reflexology. It is hypothesized that practitioner-applied reflexology would create more relaxation and thus a change in cortisol.

Outcomes from other studies (Pulse): Significant difference in pulse rate, respiratory rate, blood pressure in one session (41)*• (Healthy volunteers), (28)• (Senior citizens), (5)*^ (Cancer); Daily for 30-40 days Blood pressure, pulse rate, significant difference (30)*+ (Coronary heart disease patients); Daily for 30-40 days Pulse rate: reflexotherapy group (before): pulse rate 86-74 and (after): 76-70 (30)*+ (Coronary heart disease patients); Unknown length of time Improvement in pulse rate (7)*^ (Diabetes); Significant difference for work 1 / week for 4 weeks, 30 minutes each (31)*• (Nursing home residents)

Outcomes from other studies (Diastolic blood pressure) *See above Anxiety, Cortisol, Mealtonin.*

Outcomes from other studies (Cortisol) *See above Anxiety, Cortisol, Melatonin.*

Osteoarthritis joint pain (US)(144)*

"Osteoarthirits patients were randomly assigned to one of three groups (41 in the treatment group of foot reflexology, 39 placebo-foot massage group, and 39 control group-arthritis information) for the experimental pretest-posttest controlled clinical trial. Pain was measured before and after the 15-minute intervention. A limitation was the researcher administering all interventions and questionnaires."

Results: The groups receiving either reflexology or placebo-foot massage had significantly less posttest pain than those receiving arthritis information. "Reflexology, however, did not statistically result in less pain than massage. Clinical effect was found in the reflexology group who had 8 to 18% improvement (less pain on all pain scales), compared with those in the massage group."

Question about protocol design: Were duration (15 minute session) and frequency (one session) sufficient to create change? As noted by the researcher, both treatment and control interventions provided by the same practitioner

Post surgical recovery (Austria) (81)*

Foot reflexology or foot massage were applied following surgery 15 minutes for 5 days.

Results show that the women in the Foot Reflexology group were more able to void without problems, after the indwelling catheter had been removed than did women in the comparison groups. There was also a tendency in the Foot Reflexology group for the indwelling catheter to be removed earlier than in the other groups. In comparison the Foot Reflexology subjects slept worse than the others. Foot Massage group members showed significant results in the subjective measures of well-being, pain and sleep.

Question about design protocol: The level of pressure applied during reflexology work is unknown. Further research could determine the outcome for a lighter intensity of pressure or a generally applied reflexology technique not directed at or even avoiding foot reflex areas reflecting site of surgery.

Continued on next page.

Continued from previous page.

Outcomes from other studies: Studies on reflexology applied to post-operative pain show pain reduction: "patients who received foot reflexology treatment requires 25 to 35 percent less standard pain medication compared to the control group" (101)* (General surgery) and "The posttest mean score of pain of an experimental group was significantly lower than of a control group ... The posttest mean score of frequency pain medication taking of an experimental group was significantly lower than of a control group"(143)* (Elderly, prostatectomy). The "unpleasant symptoms score" was lowest for the foot reflexology with aroma therapy group. (106)* (Open-heart surgery)

Post-traumatic stress disorder (Northern Ireland) (133)

Foot reflexology was applied in an unknown number of sessions to the 75 study participants, victims of community violence in Northern Ireland. Results showed a significant improvements in psychological health and levels of depression over time. Changes in post-traumatic stress disorder symptom severity were not significant

Question about design protocol: Unknown number of sessions.

Outcomes from other studies: Reflexology work was applied weekly to 15 Israeli soldiers suffering from post traumatic stress disorder. Research showed relief from symptoms including anger, depression and muscle tension; Improved sleep patterns, levels of concentration and a lift in overall mood.Relief lasted 3 days. Researchers suggested reflexology work be applied 2 or 3 times a week. (132)

Chapter Eleven

Control Groups:
Impact on Outcomes

See also page 24.

> **Key**
> * Controlled study
> • PubMed (National Institute of Health)
> ^ Published in a peer-reviewed journal (Korea)
> + Published in a peer reviewed journal (China)

Control Groups: Impact on Outcomes

Placebo / Sham Reflexology Control Group	Foot Massage Control Group	Same Practitioner: Foot Massage / Reflexology	Other Control Group	Outcome	Study Details
√	√			Positive	**Cancer (Quality of life) (151)•** 100% of participants who received a 40-minute reflexology session benefitted from an improvement in 18 indexes of quality of life, significantly better than placebo reflexology group, with a 67.5% benefit. The placebo reflexology group received a gentle foot massage that did not stimulate the reflexology points. Patients were blinded to the intervention.
√				Positive	**Intestinal function (Healthy subjects) (68)*•** Significant changes in reflexology group (reflexology work on "zones assigned to the intestines") and no significant changes in placebo group (reflexology work on "zones unrelated to the intestines")
√				Positive	**Kidney function (Healthy subjects) (69)*•** Significant differences between the reflexology (work on "zones corresponding to the right kidney") and placebo groups (reflexology work on "other foot zones").
√ (Same practitioner)				Positive	Premenstrual syndrome (38)*• "significantly greater decrease in premenstrual symptoms for the women given true reflexology treatment than for the women in the placebo group"

Placebo / Sham Reflexology Control Group	Foot Massage Control Group	Same Practitioner: Foot Massage / Reflexology	Other Control Group	Outcome	Study Details
√				Positive	**Colic (138)** "In groups A and B (presumed non-effective reflexological treatment and presumed effective treatment), half the patients were "cured," which was significantly better than in group C (Control). There was no significant difference between groups A and B, but B seemed better than group A. B was significantly better than C."
√		√		Mixed	**AIDS (42)*** "Significant differences between the foot reflexology and mimic reflexology groups on the fatigue and pain intensity scale, but not on a 1-item numeric pain intensity scale."
√				Mixed	**Knee replacement (141)*** There was no significant difference (in hospital stay, long term pain killers) in any of the three groups, with the exception of significantly less morphine consumption in the early postoperative period (48 hours after surgery) in patients receiving real (light pressure reflexology) or placebo reflexology treatment (full reflexology session without areas "thought by the reflexologist to influence healing of the knee").

Placebo / Sham Reflexology Control Group	Foot Massage Control Group	Same Practitioner: Foot Massage / Reflexology	Other Control Group	Outcome	Study Details
√		Unknown		Negative	**Ovulation (164)*** The rate of ovulation during true reflexology was 11 out of 26 (42%), and during sham reflexology it was 10 out of 22 (46%). Pregnancy rates were 4 out of 26 in the true group and 2 out of 22 in the control group.
"Relaxing" vs. Lymphatic reflexology			√	Mixed	**Edema in pregnancy (148)*•** "(All groups: control: period of rest; 'relaxing' reflexology techniques; specific 'lymphatic' reflexology technique) had a non-significant oedema-relieving effect. … There was no statistically significant difference in the circumference measurements between the three groups … A 'perceived wellbeing' score revealed the lymphatic technique group significantly increased their wellbeing the most."
√ (Sham group)				Mixed	**Lower back pain (93)***"scores for pain reduced in the treatment group by a median value of 2.5 cm, with minimal change in the sham group (0.2 cm). Secondary outcome measures produced an improvement in both groups… (McGill pain questionnaire: 18 points in the reflexology group and 11.5 points in the sham group)."

Placebo / Sham Reflexology Control Group	Foot Massage Control Group	Same Practitioner: Foot Massage / Reflexology	Other Control Group	Outcome	Study Details
√				Negative	**Asthma (139)*•** "Objective lung function tests did not change. Subjective scores and bronchial sensitivity to histamine improved on both regimens but no differences were found in the groups receiving active or placebo ('simulated') reflexology."
√ (Sham nonspecific massage of the calf area)				Positive	**Multiple sclerosis (98)*** Reflexology work ("Reflexology treatment included manual pressure on specific points in the feet and massage of the calf area") showed significant improvement in alleviating motor, sensory and urinary symptoms as opposed to the control group ("nonspecific massage of the calf area"). Borderline improvement in muscle strength scores of both groups.
√ Sham TENS				Positive	**Pain threshold and tolerance (75)** Significant increase in pain tolerance and pain threshold when compared to the sham TENS group.
	√	√		Mixed	**Constipation in children (61)*** Results showed "significant differences between Reflexology and Control groups in bowel frequency and total constipation symptom score at 12 weeks; there was a significant difference between reflexology and (foot) massage for total constipation symptom score but not for bowel frequency."

Placebo / Sham Reflexology Control Group	Foot Massage Control Group	Same Practitioner: Foot Massage / Reflexology	Other Control Group	Outcome	Study Details
	√	√	√	Mixed	**Heart baroreceptors (Healthy subjects) (26)*** Significantly greater reductions in baroreceptor reflex sensitivity in the foot reflexology and foot massage groups compared to the control group, but no difference between reflexology and foot massage groups.
	√	√	√	Mixed	**Osteoarthritis (Joint pain) (144)*** Both reflexology and foot massage groups had significantly less pain than the control group (arthritis information). "Reflexology, however, did not statistically result in less pain than massage. Clinical effect was found in the reflexology group who had 8 to 18% improvement (less pain on all pain scales), compared with those in the massage group."
	√			Mixed	**Incontinence (36)*•** "There was significant change in the number of daytime frequency in the reflexology group when compared with the (foot) massage group. There was also a decrease in the 24-hour micturition frequency in both groups, but the change was not statistically significant "

Placebo / Sham Reflexology Control Group	Foot Massage Control Group	Same Practitioner: Foot Massage / Reflexology	Other Control Group	Outcome	Study Details
	√			Mixed	**Post surgical recovery (81)*** Reflexology group members were "more able to void without problems, after the indwelling catheter had been removed. There was also a tendency in the Foot Reflexology-group for the indwelling catheter to be removed earlier. In comparison the Foot Reflexology subjects slept worse than the others. Foot Massage showed significant results in the subjective measures of well-being, pain and sleep."
	√	√		Negative	**Hospice /palliative care (136)*•** Reflexology work did not show a greater effect of reflexology over simple foot massage and did not demonstrate a cumulative effect in anxiety and depression. ..."However, the symptom score showed a significant improvement in appetite and mobility for the foot massage group."
	√	√		Mixed	**Menopause (UK) (37)*•** ""Anxiety and depression scores fell in both groups to between 50% and 70% of baseline values, with a clear time effect but no significant difference between treatment (foot reflexology) and control (foot massage) groups. Similar changes were found for severity of hot flushes and night sweats."

Placebo / Sham Reflexology Control Group	Foot Massage Control Group	Same Practitioner: Foot Massage / Reflexology	Other Control Group	Outcome	Study Details
	√			Negative	**Hypertension patients (58)*** There was no statistical difference between treatment groups (reflexology and 'light foot massage without pressure on specific reflexology areas') post-intervention."
	√			Negative	**Post surgical recovery (82)*** "The simple (foot) massage turned out to be a relaxing, positive experience, whereas foot reflexology had various effects, some of them even negative. Foot reflexology is not recommended for acute, abdominal postsurgical situations in gynecology because it can occasionally trigger abdominal pain."

Bibliography

Key

* Controlled study

• PubMed (National Institute of Health

^ Published in a peer-reviewed journal (Korea)

+ Published in a peer reviewed journal (China)

(1)*^ Lee YM, "The Effects of Foot Reflexology on Depression and Anxiety in Coal Workers' Pneumoconiosis," *Korean Journal Rehabilitative Nursing* 2005 Jun; 8(1):31-37. Korean. Department of Nursing, Kangwon Tourism College. ymlee6505@hanmail.ne

(2)*•^ Lee YM, Sohng KY, "The Effects of Foot Reflexology on Fatigue and Insomnia in Patients suffering from Coal Workers' Pneumoconiosis," *Journal of Korean Academic Nursing* 2005 Dec;35(7):1221-1228. Korean. Department of Nursing, Kangwon Tourism College. ymlee6505@hanmail.net; College of Nursing, The Catholic University of Korea (PMID: 16418548)

(3)*•^ Lee YM. " Effect of Self-Foot Reflexology Massage on Depression, Stress Responses and Immune Functions of Middle Aged Women," *Journal of Korean Academic Nursing* 2006 Feb;36(1):179-188. Korean. Department of Nursing, Inje University. lym312@inje.ac.kr (PMID: 16520577)

(4)*•^ Yang JH. "The Effects of Foot Reflexology on Nausea, Vomiting and Fatigue of Breast Cancer Patients Undergoing Chemotherapy," *Journal of Korean Academic Nursing* 2005 Feb;35(1):177-185. Korean. Department of Nursing, Inje University, Korea. jhyang@inje.ac.kr (PMID: 15778569)

(5)*^ Won JS, Jeong IS, Kim JS, Kim KS.,"Effect of Foot Reflexology on Vital Signs, Fatigue and Mood in Cancer Patients receiving Chemotherapy," *Journal of Korean Academic Nursing.* 2002 Apr;9(1):16-26. Korean.Department of Nursing, Seoul Health College, Korea. Department of Nursing, College of Medicine, Pusan National University, Korea; Head Nurs of GS Dept, Dondaemoon Hospital of Ewha Woman's University, Korea; College of Nursing, Seoul National University, Korea kimks@snu.ac.kr

(6)*^ Jeong IS, "Effect of Self-Foot Reflexology on Peripheral Blood Circulation and Peripheral Neuropathy in Patients with Diabetes Mellitus," *Journal of Korean Academic Fundamental Nursing* 2006 Aug;13(2):225-234. Korean

(7)*^ Kim KS, "Effect of Foot Reflex Massage on Stress Responses, and Glucose Level of Non-Insulin Dependent Diabetes Mellitus Patients," *Korean Journal Rehabilitative Nursing* 2003 Dec;6(2):152-163. Korean.

(8)*^ Cho GY, Park HS, "Effects of 6-week Foot Reflexology on the Blood Pressure and Fatigue in Elderly Patients with Hypertension" *Journal of Korean Academic Fundamental Nursing* 2004 Aug;11(2):138-147. Korean.Department of Nursing Research Institute of Nursing Science, Pusan National University, Korea. gycho677@hanmail.net College of Medicine, Nursing Department, Pusan National University, Korea

(9)*^ Ko YS, Park MK., "Effects of Self-foot Reflexology on Fatigue and Sleep States in Women Nurses," *Korean Journal Women Health Nurs*ing 2007 Mar;13(1):21-27. Korean. Department of Nursing, Kwangyang Health College, 233-1, Dukrye-ri, Kwangyang-eup, Kwangyang-si, Chonnam, Korea. sook4095@hanmail.net Department of Nursing, Nambu University, Korea.

(10)*^ Oh SY, "The Effects of Hand Reflexology on Saeng-Chi and Immunity in ESRD Patients," *Journal of Korean Academic Fundamental Nursing* 2002 Aug;9(2):213-225. Korean. Seoul Women's College of Nursing, Korea. seiyng5@snjc.ac.kr

(11)*•^ Park HS, Cho GY, "Effects of Foot Reflexology on Essential Hypertension Patients," *Journal of Korean Academic Nursing* 2004 Aug;34(5):739-750. Korean. Department of Nursing, Pusan National University, Korea. Nursing Research Institute of Nursing Science, Pusan National University, Korea. gycho677@hanmail.net (PMID: 15502439)

(12)*^ Lee YM., "Effects of Foot Reflexology Massage on Climacteric Symptom, Fatigue and Physiologic Parameters of Middle Aged Women," *Journal of Korean Academic Nursing* 2006 Jun;18(2):284-292. Korean.Department of Nursing, Inje University, Korea. lym312@inje.ac.kr

(13)*^ Oh HS, Ahn SA., "The Effects of Foot Reflexology on Pain and Depression of Middle-aged Women with Osteoarthritis," *Korean Journal Rehabilitative Nursing* 2006 Jun;9(1):25-33. Korean. College of Nursing, Gyeong-Sang National University, JinJu, Gyeongnam, Korea. nhsoh@gshp,gsnu.ac.kr Department of Beauty Design, JinJu International University, JinJu, Gyeongnam, Korea.

(14)*^ Park SH., "Effects of Foot-Reflexology Massage on Body Weight, Lower Extremity Edema and Serum Lipids in Postpartum Women," *Korean Journal Women Health Nursing* 2007 Jun;13(2):105-114. Korean. Department of Beauty Cosmetology, Vision College of Jeonju Completion of doctor course, Korea. shiningheart@hanmail.net

(15)*^ Kim YH, Cho SH, "The Effect of Foot Reflexology on Premenstrual Syndrome and Dysmenorrhea in Female College Students," *Korean Journal Women Health Nursing*. 2002 Jun;8(2):212-221. Korean. Department of Nursing, Sun Cheon Cheong Am College, Korea

(16)*^ Jin SJ, Kim YK, "The Effects of Foot Reflexology Massage on Sleep and Fatigue of Elderly Women," *Journal of Korean Academic Nursing* 2005 Aug;17(3):493-502. Korean. Masan Samsung Medical Center. Catholic University of Pusan. ykkim@cup.ac.kr

(17)*^ Kang HS, Kim WO, Wang MJ, Cha NH., "The Effects of Self-foot Reflexology on Urinary Incontinence in Middle-aged Women," *Journal of Korean Academic Adult Nursing* 2004 Sep;16(3):482-492. Korean. College of Nursing Science, Kyung Hee University, Korea.

(18)*^ Kim KS, Sea H, Kang J, "The Effects of Community based Self-help Management Program on the Activity of Daily Life, Muscle Strength, Depression and Life Satisfaction of Poststroke Patients," *Korean Journal Rehabilitative Nursing* 2000 Jun;3(1):108-117. Korean.

(19)*^ Kim YH, Choi ES, "Effects of Foot Reflexology Education Program on Bowel Function, Anxiety and Depression in Nursing Students," *Korean Journal Women Health Nursing* 2003 Sep;9(3):277-286. Korean. Department of Nursing, Suncheon Cheongam College, Korea, College of Nursing, The Catholic University of Korea, Korea.

(21)*• Stephenson NL, Swanson M, Dalton J, Keefe FJ, Engelke M. "Partner-delivered reflexology: effects on cancer pain and anxiety," *Oncology Nursing Forum* 2007 Jan;34(1):127-32. School of Nursing, East Carolina University, Greenville, NC, USA. stephensonn@mail.ecu.edu (PMID: 17562639)

(22)• Grealish, L. Lomasney, A., Whiteman, B., "Foot Massage: A nursing intervention to modify the distressing symptoms of pain and nausea in patients hospitalized with cancer," *Cancer Nurse* 2000, June;23(3):237-43 (PMID: 10851775)

(23)*• Quattrin, R, Zanini A, Buchini S, Turello D, Annunziata D, Vidotti, C, Colobatti A, Brusagerro S, "Use of reflexology foot massage to reduce anxiety in hospitalized cancer patients in chemotherapy treatment: methodology and outcomes" *Journal of Nursing Management* 2006

Mar;14(2:96-105 Chair of Hygiene, DPMSC School of Medicine, University of Udine, Udine, Italy. r.quattrin@med.uniud.i (PMID: 1648721)

(24)• Kohara H, Miyauchi T, Suehiro Y, Ueoka H, Takeyama H, Morita T., "Combined modality treatment of aromatherapy, footsoak, and reflexology relieves fatigue in patients with cancer," *Journal Palliative Medicine*, 2004 Dec;7(6):791-6. (Department of Internal Medicine, Palliative Care Unit, National Sanyo Hospital, Yamaguchi, Japan. hkohara@bk4.so-net.ne.jp) (PMID: 15684846)

(25)*• Fuzhong Li, Peter Harmer, Nicole L. Wilson, K. John Fisher, "Healthy Benefits of Cobblestone-Mat Walking: Preliminary Findings," *Journal of Aging and Physical Activity*, 11(4), October 2003, p. 1 (PMID: 16078955)

(26)* Frankel, B. S. M., "The effect of reflexology on baroreceptor reflex sensitivity, blood pressure and sinus arrhythmia," *Complementary Therapies in Medicine*, Churchill, London, 1997, Vol. 5, pp. 80-84

(27)*^ Cho GY, Park HS, "Effects of 6-week Foot Reflexology on the Blood Pressure and Fatigue in Elderly Patients with Hypertension" *Journal Korean Academic Fundamental Nursing* 2004 Aug;11(2):138-147. Korean. Department of Nursing Research Institute of Nursing Science, Pusan National University, Korea. gycho677@hanmail.net College of Medicine, Nursing Department, Pusan National University, Korea.

(28)• Jirayingmongkol P, Chantein S, Phengchomjan N, Bhanggananda N, "The effect of foot massage (reflexology) with biofeedback: a pilot study to enhance health promotion," *Nursing Health Science*, 2002 Aug;4(Suppl):A4 (PMID: 12153420)

(29)*• Gunnarsdottir TJ, Jonsdottir H. "Does the experimental design capture the effects of complementary therapy? A study using reflexology for patients undergoing coronary artery bypass graft surgery," *Journal Clinical Nursing* 2007 Apr;16(4):777-85. School of Nursing, University of Minnesota, MN, USA and Faculty of Nursing, University of Iceland, Reykjavik, Iceland. (PMID: 17402960)

(30)*+ Zhongzheng, Li and Yuchun, Liu, "Clinical observation on Treatment of Coronary Heart Disease with Foot Reflexotherapy," *1998 China Reflexology Symposium Report*, China Reflexology Association, Beijing, pp. 38 - 41

(31)*• Nancy A. Hodgson, RN, PhD, CS1, Susan Andersen, BS2, and Heather Felker2. "Efficacy of Reflexology as a Palliative Treatment in Nursing Home Residents with Dementia: A Pilot Study" Presented at the 17th International Nursing Research Congress Focusing on Evidence-Based Practice (19-22 July 2006) (*Journal Alternative Complementary Medicine* 2008 Apr;14(3):269-75) (1) Madlyn and Leonard Abramson Center for Jewish Life, Polisher Research Institute, North Wales, PA, USA, (2) Research, Polisher Research Institute (formerly the Philadelphia Geriatric Center), Horsham, PA, USA (PMID: 18370580)

(32) Same as (3)

(33)*•+ Wang, X. M., "Type II diabetes mellitus with foot reflexotherapy," *Chuang Koh Chuang Hsi I Chief Ho Teas Chi*, Beijing, Vol. 13, Sept. 1993, pp 536-538 (First Teaching Hospital, Beijing) (PMID: 8111210)

(34)*+ Zhi-qin, Duan et. al., "Foot Reflexology Therapy Applied On Patients with NIDDM (non-insulin dependent diabetic mellitus)," *1993 China Reflexology Symposium*, p. 24

(35)*+ Ying, Ma, "Clinical Observation on Influence upon Arterial Blood Flow in the Lower Limbs of 20 Cases with Type II Diabetes Mellitus Treated by Foot Reflexology," *1998 China Reflexology Symposium Report*, China Reflexology Association, Beijing, pp. 97 - 99

(36)*• Mak HL, Cheon, WC, Wong T, Liu YS, Tong, WM, "Randomized controlled trial of foot reflexology for patients with (incontinence) symptomatic idiopathic detrusor overactivity," *International Urogynecol Journal Pelvic Floor Dysfunction* 2007 Jun;18(6):653-8, Department of Obstetrics and Gynaecology, Queen Elizabeth Hospital, Hong Kong, China. mhlj01@yahoo.com (PMID: 1700395)

(37)*• Williamson J, White A, Hart A, Ernst E., "Randomized controlled trial of reflexology for menopausal symptoms," *British Journal OG*, 2002 Sep; 109(9):1050-5)(PMID: 12269681)

(38)*• Oleson, Terry and Flocco, William, "Randomized Controlled Study of Premenstrual Symptoms Treated with Ear, Hand, and Foot Reflexology," *Obstetrics and Gynecology*, 1993;82(6): 906-11 (PMID: 8233263)

(39)*•+ Song RH, Kim do H., "The effects of foot reflexion massage on sleep disturbance, depression disorder, and the physiological index of the elderly," [Article in Korean], *Taehan Kanho Hakhoe Chi*. 2006 Feb;36(1):15-24. (Department of Nursing, Daejeon Health Science College. rhsong@hit.ac.kr.) (PMID: 16520560)

(40)* Lee CH, Oh SY, Park OS, Kwon IG, Jeong MA, Lee EA., "Effects of Hand Reflexology on Physiological Emotional Responses and Immunity in the Patients with Chronic illness; Chronic renal failure patients and Cancer patients (receiving hemodialysis)," Sungkyunkwan University, Korea. Seoul Women's College of Nursing, Korea. Samsung Medical Center, Korea

(41)*• McVicar AJ, Greenwood CR, Fewell D'Arcy V, Chandrasekharan S, Alldridge LC, "Evaluation, of anxiety cortisol and melatonin secretion following reflexology treatment: A pilot study in healthy individuals," Complementary Therapeutic Clinical Practice 2007 Aug;13(3):137-45 Institute of Health and Social Care, Anglia Ruskin University, Bishop Hall Lane, Chelmsford, Essex CM1 1SQ, UK. (PMID: 17631256)

(42)* Ounprasertpong LA., "Effect of foot reflexology on pain and fatigue in HIV/AIDS," International Conference AIDS. 2004 Jul 11-16; 15: abstract no. ThPeD7743. Ramathibodi Hospital, Mahidol University, Bangkok, Thailand (http://gateway.nlm.nih.gov?MeetingAbstracts/ 102281513.html)

(43)+ Zhi-xian, Ma and Jin-li, Zhang, "Foot Reflexology in the Treatment of Acromioclavicular Arthritis, *(19)96 Beijing International Reflexology Conference (Report)*, China Preventive Medical Association and the Chinese Society of Reflexology, Beijing, 1996, p. 55

(44)*• Petersen LN, Faurschou P, Olsen OT, Svendsen UG. "Asthma," Ugeskr Laeger. 1992 Jul 20;154(30)*+:2065-8. Ugeskr Laeger. 1993 Feb 1;155(5):329-31. Lungemedicinsk/allergologisk afdeling Y, Kobenhavns Amts Sygehus i Gentofte. (PMID: 1509577)

(45)*• McNeill JA, Alderdice FA, McMurray F., "A retrospective cohort study exploring the relationship between antenatal reflexology and intranatal outcomes," *Complementary Therapeutic Clinical Practice* 2006; 12: 119–25. (Queen's University, School of Nursing and Midwifery, Belfast, Ireland) (PMID: 16648089)

(46) Dr. Gowri Motha and Dr. Jane McGrath, "The Effects of Reflexology on Labour Outcome," Forest Gate, London, England, *Nursing Times*, Oct. 11, 1989

(47)* Zhang Changlong, "The application of foot reflexology in relieving labor pains," China Reflexology, Centre du Documentation du Groupes d'Etudes et de Recherches en Acupuncture, Registre des essais comaratifs randomises en acupuncture publies en 2000-2001, March 1 2001 (acudoc@wanado. fr) (http://www.meridiens.org/ECR/ecr2000.pdf)

(48) Sorrig, Kirsten, "Easier Births Using Reflexology, "Danish Reflexologists Association, Research Committee Report, Feb., 1995 (Originally published in the Danish daily newspaper "Burliness Tidende," July 15, 1988)

(49)*+ Rong-zhi, Wang, "An Approach to Treatment of Cerebral Palsy of Children by Foot Massage, A Clinical Analysis of 132 Cases," *(19)96 Beijing International Reflexology Conference (Report)*, China Preventive Medical Association and the Chinese Society of Reflexology, Beijing, 1996, p. 26

(50)*+ Shouqing, Gui; Changlong, Zhang and Desheng, Luo, "A Controlled Clinical Observation on Foot Reflexology Treatment for Cervical Spondylopathy," *1996 China Reflexology Symposium Report*, China Reflexology Association, Beijing, pp. 99-103

(51)*+ Shouqing, Gui; Changlong, Zhang; Jixai, Dong and Desheng, Luoof, "A Preliminary Study on the Mechanisms of Foot Reflexo-Massage; Its Effect on Free Radicals," *1996 China Reflexology Symposium Report*, China Reflexology Association, Beijing, pp. 128-135

(52)*• Sietam KS, Eriksen L, "Zone therapy of children with nocturnal enuresis," Ugeskr Laeger. 1998 Sep 21;160(39):5654-6. Danish (PMID: 9771058)

(53)*+ Jianguo, Liu and Jingshun, Zhang, "Foot Reflex Zone Massage in Recovery of Fatigue in Athletes," *1994 China Reflexology Symposium Report, China Reflexology Association*, Beijing, p. 98 (Xian City, Shan'xi, China)

(54) McCullough CA, Hughes CM, McDonough SM, "The effectiveness of acupuncture and reflexology in primary insomnia," Focus on Alternative and Complementary Therapies 2005; 10: 36

(55)*• Dr. P. Tovey, "Irritable bowel" *British Journal of General Practice* 2002 Jan;52(474):19-23Reported December 31, 2001 at http://news.bbc.co.uk/hi/english/health/newsid_1723000/17232900.stm (PMID: 11791811)

(56) Fisher DG, Berker M, "Reflexology for irritable bowel syndrome," *Focus on Alternative and Complementary Therapies* 2003; 8: 138

(57)• Stephenson N, Dalton JA, Carlson J, "The effect of foot reflexology on pain in patients with metastatic cancer," *Applied Nursing Research* 2003 Nov;16(4):284-6 (PMID: 14608562)

(58)* Somchock, Jeranut, "Effects of foot reflexology on reducing blood pressure in patients with hypertension," Flinders University, Australia, 2006

(59)*+ Yuru, Yang; Lingyun, Chao; Guangling, Meng; Scuwe, Cao; Jia-Mo, Hao and Suhui, Zhang, "Exploring the Application of Foot Reflexology to the Preventions and Treatment of Functional Constipation," *1994 China Reflexology Symposium Report*, China Reflexology Association, Beijing, p. 62

(60) Leila Ericksen, "Using reflexology to relieve chronic constipation," FDZ Research Committee *Sygeplejerksen* (Danish Journal of Nursing) 24th June 1992

(61)* J. S. Gordon, E. M. Alder, G. Matthews-Smith, Hendry, D. C. Wilson. "The effectiveness of reflexology as an adjunct to treatment in childhood idiopathic constipation: A single blind randomised controlled trial," *Archives of Disease in Childhood*: Volume 91 Supplement 1 April 2006p A13

(62)+ Bing-zhao, Zhang, "Effect of Foot Massage (Reflexology) on a Patient with Angina Observing with EKG; A Case Report," *1994 China Reflexology Symposium Report*, China Reflexology Association, Beijing, p. 53

(63) Paul Joseph, U. Rajendra Acharya, Chua, Kok Poo, Johnny Chee, Lim Choo, S. S. Iyengar, Hock Wei, "Effect of reflexological stimulation on heart rate variability," *Science Direct*, 4 February 2004

(64) Putman, J. Sunde M. (1999). "Reflexology and its effect on the EEG at C3 and C4," *Journal of Neurotherapy*, Vol. 3, No 2, 36-43.

(65)• Kannathal Natarjan, Rajendra Acharya U, Fadhilah Alias, Thelma Tiboleng and Sadasivan K. Puthusserypady, "Nonlinear analysis of EEG signals at different mental states," BioMedical Engineering OnLine, 3:7, 16 March 2004: (PMID: 15023233)

(66)• N. Kannathal, Joseph K. Paul, C. M. Lim and K. P. Chua, "Effect of Reflexology on EEG - A Nonlinear Approach," *The American Journal of Chinese Medicine*, Vol. 32, No. 4, 641-650, 2004: (PMID: 15481653)

(67)• Brown C, Ludo C, "Reflexology: A treatment plan for phantom limb pain?" *Physiotherapy* 2007;93(S1):S185 "Reflexology treatment for patients with lower limb amputations and phantom limb pain- An exploratory pilot study," *Complementary Therapies in Clinical Practice*, 2008 (14), 124-131 (PMID: 18396256)

(68)*• J, Egger I, Bodner G, Eibl G, Hartig F, Pfeiffer KP, Herold M., "Influence of reflex zone therapy of the feet on intestinal blood flow measured by color Doppler sonography," [Article in German] Forsch Komplementarmed Klass Naturheilkd. 2001 Apr;8(2):86-9. (Universitatsklinik fur Innere Medizin, Innsbruck, Austria) (Copyright 2001 S. Karger GmbH, Freiburg (Mur E, Schmidseder) (PMID:11340315)

(69)*• Sudmeier, I., Bodner, G., Egger, I., Mur, E., Ulmer, H. and Herold, M. "Anderung der nierendurchblutung durch organassoziierte reflexzontherapie am fuss gemussen mit farbkodierter doppler-sonograhpie," *Forsch Komplementarmed* 1999, Jum;6(3):129-34 (PMID: 14060981, UI: 99392031)

(70) Priya, M N and P K Sadasivan, "Dynamic reconstruction and analysis of EEG under the effect of reflexology," In World Congress on Medical Physics and Biomedical Engineering, 24-29 August 2003, Sydney, Australia, 2003

(71) Biyani A and P K Sadasivan, "Nonlinear Analysis of ECG under reflexology stimulation", In World Congress on Medical Physics and Biomedical Engineering, 24-29 August 2003, Sydney, Australia, 2003.

(72)• Degan M, Fabris F, Vanin F, Bevilacqua M, Genova V, Mazzucco M, Negrisolo A, "The effectiveness of foot reflexotherapy on chronic pain associated with a herniated disk," Prof Inferm. 2000 Apr-Jun;53(2):80-7 [Article in Italian] ULSS 12 Veneziana. (mardeg@libero.it) (PMID: 11272089)

(73) Margaret Berker, British Reflexology Association, Cardiac Unit of the Queen Elizabeth hospital, Birmingham, UK

(74)* Eriksen, Leila, "Reflexology use in (Pain Caused by) Ureter and Kidney Stone Attacks," Danish Reflexologists Association Research Committee Report, Feb. 1995 (Originally published in *Zonetherapeuten*, No. 6, 1993)

(75) Carol Samuel (Department of Pharmacy and Biomedical Sciences, University of Portsmouth, UK) "The effects on reflexology on pain threshold and tolerance in an ice-pain experiment on healthy human subject," May 13, 2007, International Congress on Complementary Medical research (Conference), www.CMR-muc2007.de

(76)+ Jin Hui, "Reflexology Applied as a Pain-Killer - Observation of 60 Cases," *1998 Beijing International Reflexology Conference Report*, China Reflexology Association, Beijing, p, 86-88

(77)* Diane G. Heatley MD, Glen E. Leverson PhD, Kari E. McConnell RN, and Tony L. Kille (the University of Wisconsin School of Medicine, Madison, WI) "Nasal Irrigation for the Alleviation of Sinonasal Symptoms," presented Monday, September 25, 2000, at the American Academy of Otolaryngology--Head and Neck Surgery Foundation Annual Meeting/Oto Expo, being held September 24-27, 2000, at the Washington, DC Convention Center; Diane G. Heatley, Kari E.

McConnell, Tony L. Kille and Glen E. Leverson, "Nasal irrigation for the alleviation of sinonasal symptoms" *Otolaryngology - Head and Neck Surgery*, Vol. 125, Issue 1, July 2001, Pages 44-48,

(78)*+ Xiaojian, Ying, "Foot Reflexology as an Accessory Treatment after External Lithotrity a Clinical Observation of 46 Cases," *1996 China Reflexology Symposium Report*, China Reflexology Association, Beijing, pp. 58 - 59

(79)+ Yue-jin, Zhang; Jing-Fang, Chung and Bao-rong, Ju, "Observation of the Effect of Foot Reflex Area Massage on 34 Cases of Calouli of Urinary Tract," *(19)96 Beijing International Reflexology Conference (Report)*, 1996, China Preventive Medical Association and the Chinese Society of Reflexology, Beijing, 1996, p. 46

(80)• Gambles M, Crooke M, Wilkinson S, "Evaluation of a hospice based reflexology service: a qualitative audit of patient perceptions," *European Journal Oncological Nursing* 2002 Mar;6(1):37-44. (Marie Curie Cancer Care, Marie Curie Centre Liverpool, Speke Road, Woolton, Liverpool, L25 8QA, UK) (PMID: 12849608)

(81)* Kesselring A., Spichiger E., Muller M, "Foot Reflexology: an intervention study," *Pflege* 1998, Aug; 11(4):213-8 (PMID: 9775925)

(82)* Kesselring A., "Foot Reflexology massage: a clinical study." Forsch Komplementarmed 1999 Feb; 6 Suppl 1:38-40 (PMID: 10077716)

(83)+ Zhi-wen, Gong and Wei-song, Xin, "Foot Reflexology in the Treatment of Functional Dyspepsia: A Clinical Analysis of 132 Cases," *(19)96 Beijing International Reflexology Conference (Report)*, China Preventive Medical Association and the Chinese Society of Reflexology, Beijing, 1996, p. 37

(84)*+ Shou-qing, Gui; Yuna-zhong, Li; Xian-qing, Xiao; Chen Shengping and Gu Xuejauna (The People's Hospital, Xianning District, Hubei Province), Zhu Shanhan, Liao Enguang (The People's Hospital of Hubei Province) and Luo Desheng (Xianning College of Medicine, Hubei Province), "Impact of the Massotherapy Applied to Foot Reflexes on Blood Fat of Human Body," *1998 China Reflexology Symposium Report*, China Reflexology Association, Beijing, pp. 34-37

(85)+ Dong Dahai, Xu Ping, Dong Congjun, Wei Lihua, "Treatment of 4 Cases of Infertility with Foot Reflexotherapy," *1998 China Reflexology Symposium Report*, China Reflexology Association, Beijing, pp. 58-59

(86)*+ Shou-qing, Gui; Xian-qing, Xiao; Yuna-zhong, Li; and Wan-yan, Fu, "Impact of the Massotherapy Applied to Foot Reflexes on Blood Fat of Human Body," *1996 China Reflexology Symposium Report*, China Reflexology Association, Beijing, p. 21

(87)*+ Gao Wa. Wang Zhen, Liu Haige, "Preliminary Exploration of Treatment for Insomnia," *1996 China Reflexology Symposium Report*, China Reflexology Association, Beijing, pp. 7-8

(88) Trousdale, Peta and Uphoff-Chmielnik, Andrea, "Making Connections, User Perception of the Effects of Reflexology & Counselling: an evaluation of a complementary health care project at Worthing Mind," September 1997

(89)+ Sun Jianhua, "Observation on the Therapeutic Effect of 82 Cases of Climacterium Syndrome (menopause) Treated with Reflexotherapy," *1998 China Reflexology Symposium Report*, China Reflexology Association, Beijing, pp. 60-61

(90)*• "Reflexology in the management of encopresis and chronic constipation," *Pedeatric Nursing*, April 2003, Vol 15 No. 3 (PMID: 12715585)
http://216.239.53.100/search?q=cache:ZbjisK7w7igJ:www.nursing-standard.co.uk/archives/pn_pdfs/pnvol15n3/pnv15n3p2021.pdf+reflexology+research+%2Bnursing&hl=en&ie=UTF-8

(91)⁺ Ji-ming, Lu, "Therapeutic Recording of a Case of Epilepsy Treated with Reflexology," *1994 China Reflexology Symposium Report*, China Reflexology Association, Beijing, p. 25 (Ningxia Reflexology Association)

(92) Brendstrup, Eva and Launsø, Laila, "Headache and Reflexological Treatment," The Council Concerning Alternative Treatment, The National Board of Health, Denmark, 1997

(93)* F. Quinna, C.M. Hughesb, and G.D. Baxter, "Reflexology in the management of low back pain: A pilot randomised controlled trial," *Complementary Therapies in Medicine*, 2007 05 011 aHealth and Rehabilitation Sciences Institute, University of Ulster, Shore Road, Newtownabbey, Co. Antrim BT37 OQB, United Kingdom: bSchool of Life and Health Sciences, University of Ulster, Shore Road, Newtownabbey, Co. Antrim BT37 OQB, United Kingdom Centre for Physiotherapy Research, School of Physiotherapy, University of Otago, Dunedin, New Zealand: Corresponding author at: School of Health Sciences, University of Ulster, Shore Road, Newtownabbey, Co. Antrim BT37 OQB, United Kingdom. Tel.: +44 28 9036 6227.

(94)* Lafuente A et al (1990). "Effekt der Reflex zonenbehandlung am FuB bezuglich der prophylaktischen Behandlung mit Flunarizin bei an Cephalea-Kopfschmerzen leidenden Patieten (migraine headache," Erfahrungsheilkunde. 39, 713-715.

(95)*+ Lingyun, Yuru, Zhao; Yang Yuru, Feng gu; Jiamo, Hao; Shuwen, Cao and Xiulan, Zhang, "Observation on Improvement of Feeble-Minded Children's Social Abilities by Foot Reflexo-Therapy," *1998 China Reflexology Symposium Report*, China Reflexology Association, Beijing, pp. 24 - 28

(96)*+ Siu-lan, Li, "Galactagogue Effect of Foot Reflexology in 217 Parturient Women (milk secretion / lactation in new mothers)," *(19)96 Beijing International Reflexology Conference (Report)*, China Preventive Medical Association and the Chinese Society of Reflexology, Beijing, 1996 p. 14

(97)* Joyce M, Richardson R., "Reflexology helps multiple sclerosis." *Journal Alternative Complementary Medicine* July 1997 10-12 (www.internethealthlibrary) (MS Centre (Glasgow), Unit 16, Chapel Hill Industrial Estate, Maryhill, Glasgow G20 9BD, Tel: 0141 945 3344)

(98)* Siev-Ner I, Gamus D, Lerner-Geva L, Achiron A," Reflexology treatment relieves symptoms of multiple sclerosis: a randomized controlled study," *Multiple Sclerosis* 2003 Aug;9(4):356-61(Complementary Medicine Clinic, Department of Orthopedic Rehabilitation, Sheba Medical Center, Tel-Hashomer, Israel) (PMID: 12926840)

(99)*+ Zhi-ming, Liu and Song, Fang, "Treatment of Neurodermatitis by Foot Reflex Area Massage (with a test group of 15 and a control group of 15)," *(19)96 Beijing International Reflexology Conference (Report)*, China Preventive Medical Association and the Chinese Society of Reflexology, Beijing, 1996, p. 16

(100) Duan Shuang-Feng. "Foot reflexology in neurosism (nervous exhaustion): Clinical Observation of 20 cases," Presented at the China Reflexology Symposium in Beijing (July 1993)

(101)* Shweta Choudhary PhD (Dept of Biophysics), Dr. Guresh Kumar, Dr. Kulwant Singh (Dept. of Biostatistics), All-India Institute of Medical Science, New Delhi, India

(102)+ Liang-cai, Pei, "Observation of 58 Infantile Pneumonia by Combined Method of Medication with Foot Massage, A Clinical Analysis of 132 Cases," *(19)96 Beijing International Reflexology Conference (Report)*, China Preventive Medical Association and the Chinese Society of Reflexology, Beijing, 1996, p. 34

(103) Lone Victoria Schumann, "Pilot Study Indicates that Reflexology has Effect On Women Suffering from Polycystic Ovaries (PCO) and Polycystic Ovary Syndrome (PCOS)," May,

2007 www.fdz.dk; Contact: Lone Victoria Schumann, Project Manager, Bentzonsvej 9, kl.th., DK-2000 Frederiksberg; lv.schumann@jubii.dk - www.schumann-zoneterapi.dk - Tel.+45 3888 7000; FDZ, Overgade 14, 1.tv., DK-5000 Odense, leme@fdz.dk - www.fdz.dk - Tel.+45 7027 8850

(104) Teruo, Nakamura, "Using Technical Measuring Machine," *RWO-SHR Health'90 Worldwide Conference Tokyo Report*, Best Care, Tokyo, pp. 45 - 54

(105)* Helen Poole, Peter Murphy, Sheila Glenn, Presented at the Annual Meeting of the American Pain Society (Treatment Approaches (Physical) E03 - Holistic/Alternative Medicine Poster #807), Published as Poole, H. M., Murphy, P., & Glenn, S. (2001) Evaluating the efficacy of reflexology for chronic back pain. *The Journal of Pain*, 2(2), 47 http://www.ampainsoc.org/abstract/2001/data/221/

(106)* Suthathip Kasedluksame, "The Effect of preoperative information combined with foot reflexology with aromatherapy on unpleasant symptoms in post opened-heart surgery patients" Thesis, 2005 Chulalongkorn University, Nursing Science, Thailand (Chanokporn jitpanya, Advisor); http://library.car.chula.ac.th:82/search*thx/?searchtype=X&searcharg=hand+reflexology&sortdropdown=-&SORT=DZ&extended=0&SUBMIT=Search&searchlimits=&searchorigarg=Xfoot+massage%26SORT%3DDZ

(107)* (Eichelberger G (1993) Study of foot reflex zone massage. Alternatives to tablets. Krankenpfiege - Soins Infirmiers. 86, 61-63) Kesselring, A. Fussrelszonemassage. Schweiz med Wonchenschr suppi (Switzerland) 1994, 62, pp. 88-93

(108) Bauneholm School of Reflexology, Denmark

(109)+ Zhou Xin, Zhou Gengye, "Treatment of Prostatic Hypertrophy (frequent, urgent, difficult and nocturnal urination) with Reflexotherapy," *1998 China Reflexology Symposium Report*, China Reflexology Association, Beijing, pp. 50-55

(110)*+ Xiao-li, Chen, "Hyperplasia of Prostate Gland Treated by Foot Reflex Area Health Promoting Method (as tested by Ultrasonographic examinations)," *1996 China Reflexology Symposium Report*, China Reflexology Association, Beijing, October 1996, pp. 32 - 33

(111)+ Yue-jin, Zhang; Jing-Fang, Chung and Bao-rong, Ju, "Observation of the Effect of Foot Reflex Area Massage on 34 Cases of Calouli of Urinary Tract," *(19)96 Beijing International Reflexology Conference (Report)*, 1996, China Preventive Medical Association and the Chinese Society of Reflexology, Beijing, 1996, p. 46

(112)*+ Yu-lian, Zao, "Clinical Observation on Treatment of Infection of Urinary Tract by Foot Massage," *(19)96 Beijing International Reflexology Conference (Report)*, China Preventive Medical Association and the Chinese Society of Reflexology, Beijing, 1996, p. 17

(113)*+ Cailian, Lin, "Clinical Observation on Treatment of 40 Cases of Uroschesis with Reflexology," *1998 China Reflexology Symposium Report*, China Reflexology Association, Beijing, pp. 52 - 53

(114)+ Gongcheng, Shen, "Treatment of Herpes Zoster with Foot Reflex Zone Massage," *1996 China Reflexology Symposium Report*, China Reflexology Association, Beijing, 1996, p. 83-85

(115)*+ Zhensheng, Wu, "Observation on the Therapeutic Effect of 15 Cases of Gout treated with Foot Reflexotherapy," *1996 China Reflexology Symposium Report*, China Reflexology Association, Beijing, 1996, pp. 104-109

(116)*+ Zhaoyi, Xu, "Clinical Observation on the Treatment for 83 Cases with Cervical Spondylosis by Hand Massage (Reflexology) Combined with Tui-na," *1996 China Reflexology Symposium Report*, China Reflexology Association, Beijing, 1996, pp 110-114

(117)+ Zhixian, Zhao, Gengye, Zhou, Xin, Zhou, "Foot Reflexology in the Treatment for 5 Cases with Drug Toxic Deafness (Loss of Hearing)," *1996 China Reflexology Symposium Report*, China Reflexology Association, Beijing, 1996, pp.119-121

(118)+ Sheng-Chang, Tong, "Using Foot Massotherapy to Cure (4 Cases of) Hepatitis B," *1994 China Reflexology Symposium Report*, p. 70 (Guangxi Health Cadre Institute)

(119)+ Zhensheng, Wu; Xizhen, Li; Weiyu, Lu; Huixin, You; Dali, Dai; "Reflexology in Treating Adolescent Myopia: Observation of 34 Cases," *1994 China Reflexology Symposium Report*, p. 70 (Guangxi Health Cadre Institute)

(120)+ Shisheng, Wu, "Effect of Foot Massage (Sandals) on Blood Circulation," *1994 China Reflexology Symposium Report*, p. 70 (Guangxi Health Cadre Institute)

(121)*+ Ya-zhen, Xu, "Treatment of Leukopenia (low white blood cell count) with Reflexotherapy," *1998 China Reflexology Symposium Report*, China Reflexology Association, Beijing, pp. 32-33

(122)+ Dr. Gui Shouqing, Chen Shengpeng, Yang Danwei, Su Kun, Lin Jing, "Treatment of 45 Cases of Arteriae Vertebralis Type of Cervical Spondylopathy with Reflexolotherapy," *1998 China Reflexology Symposium Report*, China Reflexology Association, Beijing, pp. 79-81

(123)+Ling, Zhang, "Treatment of 29 Cases with Myopia by Foot Reflexology," *1998 China Reflexology Symposium Report*, China Reflexology Association, Beijing, pp. 84-85

(124)+ Feng Jinqi, Fan Chunmei, Feng Xingqian, "Exploration on the Effects of Pulse, Respiration and Oxygen Saturation of Blood by Different Strength of Stimulus," *1998 China Reflexology Symposium Report*, China Reflexology Association, Beijing, pp. 94-96

(125)+ Wu Zhen-sheng, Li Xue-zhen, "Treatment of 38 Cases of Ischemic Apoplexy (Stroke) with Reflexology," *1998 China Reflexology Symposium Report*, China Reflexology Association, Beijing, pp. 1-4

(126)+ Xu Ya-zhen, "Treatment of 38 Cases of Children Enuresis by Foot Massage," *(19)96 Beijing International Reflexology Conference (Report)*, 1996, China Preventive Medical Association and the Chinese Society of Reflexology, Beijing, 1996, p. 29

(127) Tang Annie M., Li Geng., Chan C.C., Wong K.K.K., Li R. and Edward Yang, "Brain Activation at Temporal Lobe Induced by Foot Reflexology: an fMRI Study," 11th Annual NeuroImage Meeting. 2005, 1445. (Publication No.102229) www.humanbrainmapping.org

(128) Tang M.Y., Li G., Chan C.C., Wong K.K.K., Li R. and Yang E.S., "Vision Related Reflex Zone at the Feet: An fMRI Study," 11th Annual NeuroImage Meeting. 2005, 1431. (Publication No. 1102226)

(129) Annie M. Tang, Geng Li, Edward S. Yang, "Comparison of Foot Reflexology and Electro-Acupuncture: An fMRI study," The Jockey Club MRI Centre, The University of Hong Kong, Pokfulam, Hong Kong 474 TH-PM; Presented at Twelfth Annual Meeting of the Organization for Human Brain Mapping www.humanbrainmapping.org; NeuroImage 31 (2006) 237

(130) Testa, Gail W., "A Study on the Effects of Reflexology on Migraine Headaches," August 2000 (Full article: http://members.tripod.com/GTesta/Dissertation11.htm

(131) *Same as (150)*

(132) Meier Teichman, PhD (Clinical Psychologist and Head of Tel Aviv's University's Bob Shapell Scholl of Social Work) and Scmuel Zaidel, "Experimental Treatment in Reflexology with Severe, Chronic Post Traumatic Stress Disorder," Institute of Human Ecology

(132a)"Reflexology On the Front Lines of Health Care (Use in post traumatic stress syndrome by soldiers in Israel)", *Massage Magazine*, November/December 1998

(133) Dillenburger, Karola, Fargas, Montserrat, Akhonzada, Rym, "Evidence-Based Practice: An Exploration of the Effectiveness of Voluntary Sector Services for Victims of Community Violence (Reflexology and other modalities used for post traumatic stress in Northern Ireland)," *British Journal of Social Work*, August 9, 2007; Correspondence to Dr. Karola Dillenburger, School of Sociology, Social Policy and Social Work, The Queen's University of Belfast, 6 College Park, Belfast B17 1LP, N. Ireland. E-mail: k.dillenburger@qub.ac.uk

(134)• Stephenson, N. L., Weinrich, S. P. and Tavakoli, A. S., "The effects of foot reflexology on anxiety and pain in patients with breast and lung cancer," *Oncology Nursing Forum*. 2000, Jan.-Feb.;27(1):67-72 (PMID:10660924)

(135) "Reflexology to improve children's aggressive and anti-social behavior to allow mainstreaming," BUD, Therapies for Life, Accessible complementary therapies for vulnerable children and adults to improve quality of life (http://www.bud-umbrella.org.uk/service.html)

(136)*• Ross, C S., Hamilton, J, Macrae, G, Docherty, C, Gould, A, Cornbleet, M A (2002). "A pilot study to evaluate the effect of reflexology on mood and symptom rating of advanced cancer patients," *Palliative Medicine* 16: 544-545 (PMID: 12465705)

(137) "Physiological Measurements for Reflexology Foot Massage," Yoshio MACHI1, Chao LIU1 and Maki FUJITA21 Dept. of Electronic Engineering, Tokyo Denki University (Tokyo, JAPAN) 2 Japan Reflexology Association Maki Fujita Reflexology School (Tokyo, JAPAN)

(138) Författare: Bennedbaek O, Viktor J, Carlsen KS, Roed H, Vinding H, Lundbye-Christensen S., "Originalets titel: Infants with colic. A heterogeneous group possible to cure? Treatment by pediatric consultation followed by a study of the effect of zone therapy on incurable colic," Publicerad: Ugeskr Laeger 2001 Jul 2;163(27):3773-8). Article published in Danish.(Institution: Aalborg Universitet, Institut for Matematiske Fag

(139)*• Brygge T, Heinig JH, Collins P, Ronborg SM, Gehrchen PM, Hilden J, Heegaard S, Poulsen LK, "Zone Therapy and Asthma," Ugeskr Laeger, 2002, Apr. 29; 164(18):2405-10- Danish language (PMID: 12024846)

(140)• Gwen K. Wyatt, Sharon Kozachik, Charles W. Given, Barbara Given, "Outcomes of Complementary Therapy Use by Cancer Patients and Family Members," Midwest Nursing Research Society Conference, 2003; *Cancer Nurs*. 2006 Mar-Apr;29(2):84-94. School of Nursing, Johns Hopkins University, Baltimore, MD 21205, USA. skozach1@son.jhmi.edu (PMID: 16565617)

(141)* Evans SL, Nokes LDM, Weaver P, et al. "Effect of reflexology treatment on recovery after total knee replacement," *Journal Bone Joint Surgery* (British Vol) 1998;80(Suppl. 2):172

(142)*+ Hui-xian, Duanmu, "A Clinical Analysis of Foot Reflexomassage for Treatment of 45 Cases with Infantile Asthma," *1994 China Reflexology Symposium Report*, China Reflexology Association, Beijing, October 1994, pp. 41 - 43 (Health Center for Women and Children, Haimen, Jiangsu Province, China)

(143)* Tanyakhanok Pongpiyapibon, "Effects of symptom management with reflexology program on pain and frequency of pain medication taking in elderly patient with prostatectomy" Thesis, 2005, Chulalongkorn University, Nursing Science, Thailand (Sirphan Sasat, Advisor)

(144)* Laree J Schoolmeesters PhD, RN, "The Effect of Reflexology on Self-Reported (Osteoarthritis) Joint Pain," Southern Nursing Research Society Proceedings: 2007 Annual Conference, Feb 22, 2007

(145)• Baerheim A, Algroy R, Skogedal KR, Stephansen R, Sandvik H, "Feet - a diagnostic tool?" Tidsskr Nor Laegeforen 1998 Feb 20;118(5):753-5 (PMID: 9528375) (Norwegian)

(146) A. White, J. Williamson, Hart A, Ernst E, "A blinded investigation into the accuracy of reflexology charts," *Complementary Therapy Medicine*, 8, 2000: 166-7

(147) Raz I, Rosengarten Y, Carasso R, (Faculty of Medicine, Faculty of Health Sciences, Ben Gurion University of the Negev) "Correlation study between conventional medical diagnosis and the diagnosis by reflexology (non conventional)," (Article in Hebrew), Harefuah, 2003 Sep;1(42)*(8-9):600-5, 646) (PMID: 14518162)

(148)*• Mollart l., "Single Blind trial addressing the differential effects of two reflexology techniques versus rest, on ankle and foot oedema in late pregnancy," *Complementary Therapeutic Nursing Midwifery*, 2003 Nov;9(4):203-8 See http://www.midwiferytoday.com/enews/enews0307.asp PMID: 14556770

(149)*• Iain S. A. Wilkinson, Samantha Prigmore and Charlotte F. Rayner Corresponding author. (St George's Hospital, Tooting, London SW17, UK; North Hampshire Hospital, Aldermaston Road, Basingstoke RG24 9NA, UK, "A randomised-controlled trail examining the effects of reflexology of patients with chronic obstructive pulmonary disease (COPD)," *Complementary Therapies in Clinical Practice*, 2005 (PMID: 16648092)

(150) Boyd, Denise, "Using reflexology: A feasibility study," *Mental Health Nursing*. Nov/Dec 2001. FindArticles.com. 03 Jan. 2008. http://findarticles.com/p/articles/mi_qa3949/is_200111/ai_n9007476 *Same as 132*

(151)• Hodgson, H. "Does reflexology impact on cancer patients' quality of life?," Apr. 2000, *Nursing Standard*, 14, 31, pp. 33-38 (PMID: 11973949)

(152)* Kim Myung Ae, Kim Su Jung, Kim Su Jin, Kim Yang Ji,(Keimyung University College of Nursing, Korea) "Effects of Hand Reflexology on Fatigue and Emotional State in Cancer Patients Receiving Radiotherapy," Article 8, Science nursing commandment No. 1, 2004. pp. 39-47

(153) Liang Jian, "Reflexology therapy for 50 patients with chronic fatigue syndrome," (Beijing Traditional Chinese Medicine Hospital Beijing 100010) Medical Information in China in July 2003 magazine article 10 paragraph 7 Vol.

(154) "Reflexology Research into Enuresis Nocturna / Bedwetting 1 & 2," Krogsgaard, Dorte; Poulsen, Edith; Kyhl, Torben; Bo Lund, Jens; and, Eriksen, Leila

(155) R.K.F. Ho, K.K. Yu, Y.Y. Tse, J.C.F. Ho, F.S.Y. Wong, Y.L. Cheng, A.W.Y. Yu, "Effectiveness of foot reflexology on cramp in hemodialysis patients" Renal Unit, Alice Ho Miu Ling, Nethersole Hospital, Hong Kong. Hong Kong Society of Nephrology, The 20th Annual Scientific Meeting, November 28, 2004, Hong Kong

(156)*+ Ma Dongmei, CAO Hui-min, Duan Feng-lian, "Foot Massage therapy reflection of the impact of peptic ulcer patients; Influence of foot massage reflection therapy on peptic ulcer patients," *Nursing Research*, 2006 22

(157)* Tsay, Shiow-Luan PhD, RN; Chen, Hsiao-Ling MS, RN; Chen, Su-Chiu MS, RN; Lin, Hung-Ru PhD, RN; Lin, Kuan-Chia PhD, "Effects of Reflexotherapy on Acute Postoperative Pain and Anxiety Among Patients With Digestive Cancer," *Cancer Nursing*. 31(2):109-115, March/April 2008.

(158)*+ Wang Cui Cheng Rui Dan, Cai Rong-hua, Chin Chu, "Reflexology bamboo (stepping) massage for the treatment of cancer chemotherapy-induced nausea and vomiting effect of ...," *Modern Nursing in 2007*, 33

(159)*+ Peng Guizhi, Liao Tao, Meng Li-fang, Wang Yuan-, Wei Jihong, Qiu snow-sheung, Wei Dan He, Zhou Ying, "Study for the effect of recovery for puerperium women treated Chinese native medicine foot bath combined with full foot bottom massage," Nurse education magazine, 2007 23

(160)*+ Zhongcuifang, Huang Lihong, HE Miao East, Zhou, Wen-Cheng Peng Pai, Hsiao-Hui Lee, Bao Jinlian, paragraph Fortunately, Wen-Jie Li, "Foot Massage on postpartum urinary system rehabilitation research," *Maternal and Child Health Care of China*, 2003, No. 09

(161)*+ Peng Guizhi, Qiu snow-sheung, Meng Li-fang, Zhou Ying, Wei Dan He, "Post-natal care and intervention on anxiety, depression impact study," *China's Health* (medical research) 2007 14

(162)*+ Yuqi, Shao-ying, Ms Aw gold, "Touch with reflexology massage on the area of weight premature infants," Zhejiang Chinese magazine 2006 02

(163)*+ Zhou Xiaoqing Zhou Xiaoqin, Zhou Xiaoqing, "Foot after cesarean section on the recovery of gastrointestinal function; the Influence of Foot Soaking and Massage on the Recovery of Digestive System after Cesarean," Contemporary nurses (Academic Edition) *Today Nurse* 2004, Section 01

(164)* Holt J, Lord J, Acharya U, White A, O'Neill N, Shaw S, Barton A., "The effectiveness of foot reflexology in inducing ovulation: a sham-controlled randomized trial." *Fertil Steril.* 2008 Jun 18. PMID: 1856552 South Devon School of Reflexology, Morningside, Loddiswell, Devon, United Kingdom.

(165)* Clausen J, Møller E. En randomiseret undersøgelse af zoneterapi ved inerti og retentio placentae (A randomised (blinded, controlled) trial of reflexology in inertia during labor). Århus Kommunehospital Afd Y8, 1992.(Reported by Andrew Vickers and Catherine Zollman ABC of complementary medicine: Massage therapies BMJ 1999; 319: 1254-1257)

(166) Kurumi Tsuruta, Hifumi Kusaba, Miyuki Yamada, Tazuko Murakata, Rika Nakatomi, "Program (bamboo stepping, stretching, rhythmic exercise) for family members with hospitalized child," *Pediatric Nursing*, July-August, 2005

(167) Makereth, Peter A., Booth, Katie, Hillier, Valerie, and Caress, Ann-Louise, "Reflexology and progressive muscle relaxation training for people with multiple sclerosis: A crossover trial," *Complementary Therapies in Clinical Practice*, Oct 2008

(168)* Sharpe D, Walker AA, Walker V, Green V, Alexandropoulos A (Institute of Rehabilitation Oncology Health,Centres, University of Hull, Hull,UK), "The Psychoneuroimmunological Effects of Reflexology in Women with Early Breast Carcinoma," *Psycho-Oncology* 15: S1 – S478 (2006) (Abstracts of the 8th World Congress of Psycho-Oncology 16th–21st October 2006 Ferrara, Venice, Italy)

(169) Nakamaru T, Miura N, Fukushima A, Kawashima R. (Tohoku University School of Medicine, Sendai, Japan; Department of Functional Brain Imaging, Institute of Development, Aging and Cancer (IDAC), Tohoku University, Sendai, Japan.) "Somatotopical relationships between cortical activity and reflex areas in reflexology: A functional magnetic resonance imaging study," Neuroscience Lett. 2008 Oct 14 PMID: 18938220

(170) Li CY, Chen SC, Li CY, Gau ML, Huang CM, "Randomised controlled trial of the effectiveness of using foot reflexology to improve quality of sleep amongst Taiwanese postpartum women,"*Midwifery.* 2009 Jul 3. (Department of Nursing, Tri-Service General Hospital, No. 325, Sec.2, Cheng-Gong Rd., Neihu, Taipei 114, Taiwan, ROC).

(171) Kim, Kyung-Mi, "The Effects of Foot Reflexology on Patients in the Remission State pf Thyroid Disease," The Graduate School of Public Health, Inje University (http://www.reportworld.co.kr/paper/view.html?no=10029778&pr_rv=rv_relate_view)

(172) Caption (Sei Young Oh), hahyejeong (Hyae Chung Ha), yiyoungsun (Young Soon Lee), Kim DS (Dong Soo Kim), yimyeongsuk (Myung Sook Lee),"The Effect of Hand Reflexology on Pain, Skin Temperature and Nursing Practice," *Korea Journal of Nursing Education*, 12, 2 Korea, Overall: 9 pages, start pages: 178 pages, January 2006

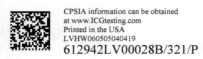

CPSIA information can be obtained
at www.ICGtesting.com
Printed in the USA
LVHW060505040419
612942LV00028B/321/P